"Newman follows the tradition of the earlier pioneers such as Dick-Read, Lamaze, and Bradley in offering practical and ground-breaking solutions to the stresses of birth, but exceeds their efforts by a wide margin. This is essential reading for birth and other professionals who handle birth-related impacts such as pediatricians, pre- and perinatal practitioners, childbirth educators, doulas, midwives, nurses, and others. It is essential reading for expectant parents who can promote the health of their babies and prevent unnecessary negative impacts via Calm Birth. And the book is magnificant reading!"

—William Emerson, Ph.D., author of more than thirty pre- and perinatal publications, and director of the Emerson Training Seminars

"Robert Newman's *Calm Birth* program provides couples and professionals alike a beautiful map, a method and a philosophy, to prepare for birth in a way that honors and helps them connect with their deepest innate nature and abilities. Meditation methods in *Calm Birth* open up a vista of hope, empowerment, inner wisdom, and confidence to trust the ability to birth naturally. Families' stories gracefully illuminate how *Calm Birth* ignites transformational experience in life, pregnancy, birth, and beyond. I hope you read this book."

—Wendy Anne McCarty, Ph.D., R.N., author of *Welcoming Consciousness* (2005) and founding chair of the Prenatal and Perinatal Psychology Program at the Santa Barbara Graduate Institute

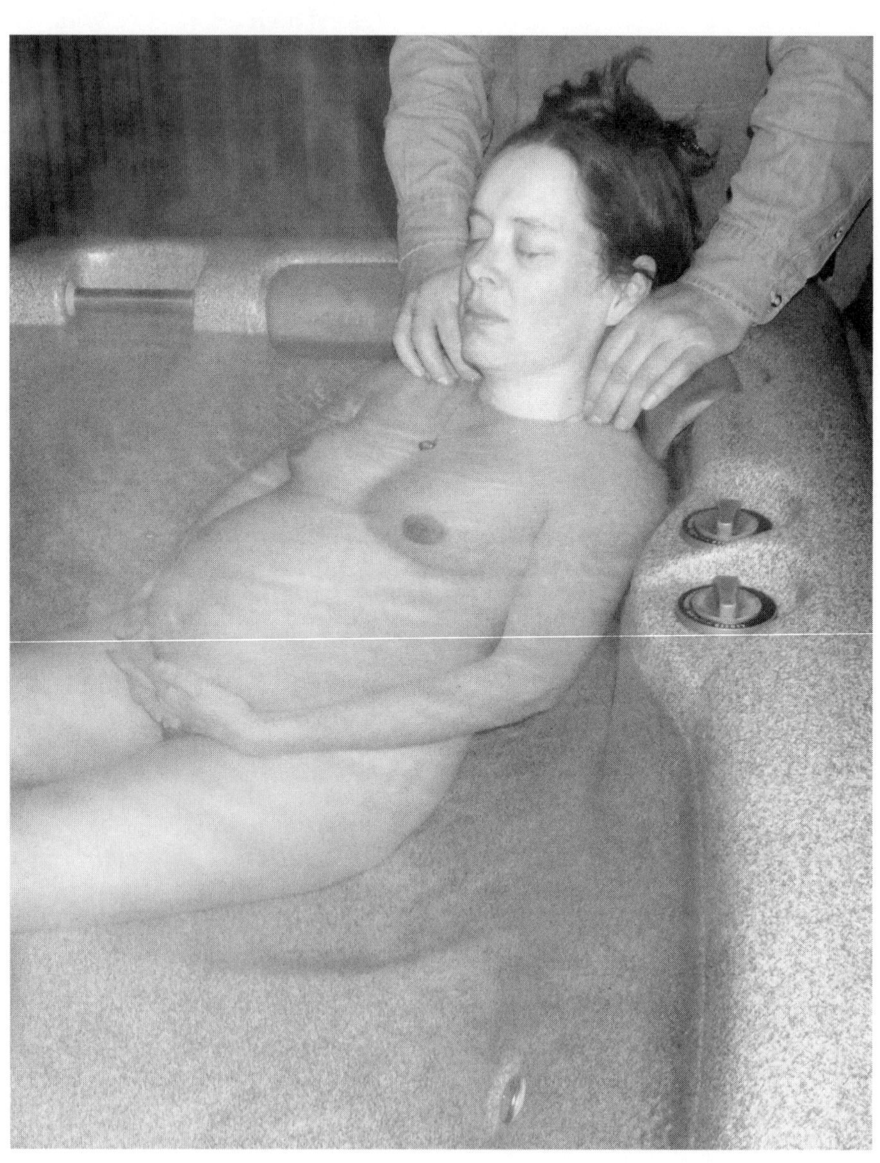

Calm Birth

New Method for Conscious Childbirth

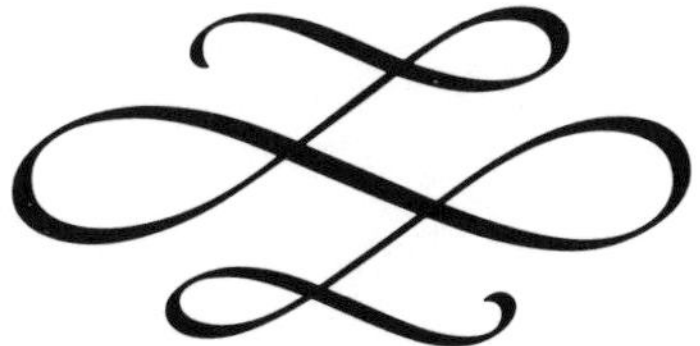

Robert Bruce Newman

Foreword by David B. Chamberlain, Ph.D.

Afterword by Ruth L. Miller, Ph.D.

North Atlantic Books
Berkeley, California

Published by
North Atlantic Books
P.O. Box 12327
Berkeley, California 94712

Interior photos by Patti Ramos
Cover and book design by Paula Morrison

Printed in the United States of America
Distributed to the book trade by Publishers Group West

Calm Birth: New Method for Conscious Childbirth is sponsored by the Society for the Study of Native Arts and Sciences, a nonprofit educational corporation whose goals are to develop an educational and crosscultural perspective linking various scientific, social, and artistic fields; to nurture a holistic view of arts, sciences, humanities, and healing; and to publish and distribute literature on the relationship of mind, body, and nature.

North Atlantic Books' publications are available through most bookstores. For further information, call 800-337-2665 or visit our website at www.northatlanticbooks.com. Substantial discounts on bulk quantities are available to corporations, professional associations, and other organizations. For details and discount information, contact our special sales department.

Library of Congress Cataloging-in-Publication Data

Newman, Robert Bruce, 1935–
Calm birth : new method for conscious childbirth / by Robert Bruce Newman ; foreword by David B. Chamberlain ; afterword by Ruth L. Miller.
p. ; cm.
Includes bibliographical references.
Summary: "Presents a childbirth methodology that combines three mind/body practices to create a prenatal and natal experience that is empowering for mother and child"—Provided by publisher.
ISBN 1-55643-612-2 (pbk.)
1. Natural childbirth. 2. Mind and body.
[DNLM: 1. Natural Childbirth—methods. 2. Meditation—methods. WQ 152 N554c 2005] I. Title.

RG661.N49 2005
618.4'5—dc22

2005025143

1 2 3 4 5 6 7 8 9 UNITED 10 09 08 07 06 05

Table of Contents

Foreword

By David B. Chamberlain, Ph.D.

IF YOU HAVE WATCHED any of the many depictions of childbirth created by Hollywood in recent years, you will quickly appreciate they are anything but calm. Catering to our worst fears (men's fears as well as women's), birth is presented as a frantic flight from home to hospital, all participants in a state of high anxiety, trying desperately to avoid a direct confrontation with a natural human function. The idea is that if we can just make it to the hospital, professionals will gladly take over and save us from ourselves!

What explains the perpetuation of these birth scripts? Probably not ignorance. Can anyone believe the screenwriters of recent generations missed out on Lamaze classes? Where else could they have learned to include those scenes where nurses are shouting at mothers to start panting at the peak of labor? No, I suspect screenwriters of making a caricature of birth for their own selfish purpose—to get laughs—while exploiting a host of subliminal fears of birth in the public at large. In doing so, writers keep stripping away the promising but fragile qualities of dignity and triumph in childbirth. But this is not a new problem.

The struggle for dignity and triumph in childbirth has had the longest possible history: since we have been reproducing ourselves as humans. For nearly all of that time, birth was a woman's business, usually in association with other women who channeled the birth wisdom of their ancestors and peers. Birth at home was from the beginning the norm for families around the globe. Although cultures and subcultures of the world continue to exert some small influence on the privacy of birth, even Eastern civilizations have largely copied the Western model of birth as a medical-surgical ritual held in hospitals. It is the new reality.

Preparation for childbirth today suffers the temblors and aftershocks of revolutionary developments in the 20th century that greatly obscured the previous culture of normal, family-centered birthing. In the United States, the Golden Age of industrialization and galloping technology brought new prominence to all medical specialties, advantaged in an unprecedented way by newly invented insurance entities. As a consequence, by the 1940s, more people were being born in hospitals than were being born at home—an epic turning point. Currently about 99 percent of U.S. births take place in hospitals.

Redefined as a medical problem, birth care changed hands from mainly women helpers to mainly men helpers; high-tech came to mean low-touch as personal care became submerged in the "active management" of birth. Importantly, basic responsibilities quickly shifted from parents to medical specialists.

The strain of this rapid transition manifests itself today in pervasive litigation between patients and doctors, chronic escalation of medical fees, and, occasionally, the failure of the insurance entities that led to industrialized medicine. Families struggle to pay the increasing costs of childbirth. Other signs of cultural exhaustion include the retreat of obstetricians from delivery of babies to the less litigious practice of gynecology, the disinterest of medical graduates in obstetrics training residencies, and the sharp drop-off of applications of college students to medical school.

In the United States and many other parts of the world, childbirth—as a natural ability of women—is besieged or abandoned. On this side of the Atlantic a natural birth in a hospital setting is a rare achievement of well-informed, well-prepared, and determined women who have found the professional support they need. Paradoxically, on the other side of the Atlantic, "normal birth" is now the goal of collaboration between the British Parliament, the National Childbirth Trust, the Royal College of Midwives, and the

Royal College of Obstetricians and Gynecologists! Cultural anthropologist Sheila Kitzinger reports that an All Party Parliamentary Group (APPG) has invited all maternity units in all regions of England to compete for two awards to be presented at the House of Commons by the Health Minister: the "Increasing Normal Births" Award and the "Most Improved Home Birth Rate" Award!

In America, where there are no such signs of support from large institutions for childbearing families, the best hope lies in inspired women taking responsibility for themselves. Childbirth is, after all, a unique ability of women, an intimate activity that abhors strangers, resists authorities, and avoids massive buildings, preferring privacy in a free and friendly environment. Importantly, it is mothers and fathers who choose both the birthplace and the helpers they want. They need options.

History is teaching us that childbearing has more viability and integrity when parents bear the central responsibility for reproduction from start to finish: choosing to conceive, communicating with the womb baby, fortifying and preparing themselves through pregnancy, deciding on the quality of birth they seek, and learning enough to give truly informed consent when dealing with professional helpers.

Surveys of mothers' satisfaction with their childbirth experiences regularly show that high on their scale of values is being cared for by people they know (not by a series of strangers), people who listen to and respect their feelings (not those who manipulate or take control of them), and, perhaps most of all, having helpers who will earnestly assist them to fulfill their personal goals for childbirth. Today, dignity and triumph in childbirth will likely require the full cooperation and respect of family-invited medical experts, midwifery experts, childbirth educators, and doulas. Of these, the "oldest profession" is, of course, midwifery, the women with birth wisdom who always presided over birth until medical specialists gained hegemony only in the last sixty years.

Childbirth educators are professionals of the 20th century, born out of the challenges and complexities of medicalized birth. Doulas, who are present in increasing numbers at birth today, have similarly evolved in relation to birth in hospitals. I see them as taking the role of trusted friends and family who were always present at home birth, but not as practitioners; they have one purpose, to give steadfast attention and support to the laboring mother. All four specialists bring valuable and distinctive gifts and all four serve "at will," that is, at the will of the parents.

Into the current mix of cultural uncertainties surrounding birth, a new form of childbirth preparation is making its entrance, appropriately named Calm Birth. The innovative program is the brainchild of Robert Newman, a longtime student and teacher of meditation and a serious reader in the field of prenatal and perinatal psychology and health. Calm Birth gives women and birth professionals practical means to improve the quality of childbirth. Like the venerable educational programs inspired by Dr. Grantly Dick-Read beginning in England in 1933, by Dr. Fernand Lamaze imported from France in the 1950s, and by Dr. Robert Bradley starting in America in 1965, Calm Birth seeks to empower women for natural childbirth and offers ideas and practical methods for them to succeed. Like the previous programs Calm Birth recognizes the central challenge posed by fear and pain, though its solution is different, and it recognizes the importance of breathing, though it teaches a form of blended breathing into both the energy body and physical body, reflecting a new vision of childbirth anatomy.

Historically, the Calm Birth program was developed by Medi-Grace, founded in 1991 by Robert Newman with Drs. John Sutton and Craig Spaniol of NASA to research and develop methods of energy medicine and mind/body medicine. The first fruit of this collaboration was *Calm Healing: Medical Uses of Meditation.* Based on successful programs of the Harvard Medical School and the University of Massachusetts Medical Center, Calm Healing trainings have been presented more than sixty times in medical centers and hospitals. Note the CD *Calm Healing: Advanced Health Care,* MG3.

The pilot program for Calm Birth began in 1998 in medical centers in Southern Oregon. The path created by the earlier successful programs opened the door for Calm Birth, now being welcomed in medical centers and hospitals in Oregon, California, and Washington.

The new program teaches a set of practices with ancient roots, assuring that what is freshly crafted has already stood the test of time. Calm Birth works with both physical anatomy and energy body anatomy, drawing on quantum physics and meditation science to access energies that are invisible but very much present. Likewise, breathing is more than physical, adding appreciation of new childbirth anatomy and potential.

At the core of the Calm Birth curriculum presented in this book are three practices that are well articulated in audioguides (for example, the CD *Calm Birth: Empowering Preparation for Childbirth,* CB3) that accompany the training. The helpfulness of these tools is acclaimed by mothers and fathers who have used them. The three practices are: the *Practice of Opening, Womb Breathing,* and *Giving and Receiving.* A brief description here will suggest how different these methods are from current models of childbirth preparation.

The *Practice of Opening* is a reclining form of progressive relaxation, a classic process of self-care made famous by Dr. Edmund Jacobson in the 1920s and 1930s. Designed to be used during the whole period of childbirth preparation, it facilitates communication between mother, father, and the unborn child. The script focuses attention on cellular life forces on a journey through the body releasing stress and reconditioning the nervous system for relaxed, harmonious functioning. Relaxation is understood to provide a gain of energy that feeds optimum development of the child. During the exercise there is a conscious alignment of the awareness of the parents with the awareness of the child—a recognition that has been missing in childbirth education.

Womb Breathing is a "sitting" meditation of twenty minutes designed for the pregnant woman and for husbands who choose to share in it. Founded on the ancient Tibetan practice of deep energy breathing, it is designed to absorb vital energy from the air to nourish both mother and child. In Calm Birth it is utilized for release of fear in contractions. Visualization is a strong component of *Womb Breathing* focusing on the physical body and energy body as one form participating in a universal energy field—ancient ideas that are now being increasingly grounded in scientific research. Visualized are energy channels ranging in size from the large central channel with its radiant series of power centers *(chakras)* to a host of small, fine conduits. Energy body anatomy can be discerned as early as the first two weeks of embryonic development; some authorities see this as a manifestation of the seamless intelligence system at work from before conception.

The third major practice, called *Giving and Receiving,* is a method of healing that can be used throughout pregnancy, in labor and delivery, in postnatal care, or at any other challenging time. Instead of taking in vital energy, as in *Womb Breathing,* you take in the energy of any adverse condition in yourself, your child, or someone else, dissolve it in natural light in your cells, and send out healing energy. This versatile method of transformation can be used for pain, illness, conflict, emotional upsets in everyday life, and to heal any residue of trauma from your own birth. Energies of intention and visualization are brought together in this act of compassion. In the process, the recipient, mother, and baby are all blessed. In ancient times, it was called "the holy secret."

From my perspective of studies in prenatal psychology, Calm Birth is arriving at an opportune time in the early years of the 21st century when, at last, the 19th-century ideas about babies (and mothers) that prevail in both medicine and psychology are finally collapsing under the weight of new evidence. An age of belief in brain matter as the sole measure of a person is giving way to a new paradigm of awareness or consciousness as the real measure of who we are.

Under the old paradigm of medicine—and childbirth education—even a full-term baby was a creature of inadequate brain, unable to sense pain or pleasure, to have true emotion, or to think, remember, or learn anything from prenatal or perinatal experience. The luxury of that dark view permitted medical doctors to concentrate entirely on physical matters and to ignore baby awareness, psyche, or self.

All three of the medical doctors who laid the foundations for childbirth education as we know it (Drs. Dick-Read, Lamaze, and Bradley) lived in that paradigm. So did the obstetricians delivering babies, and the pediatricians who invented neonatal intensive care. Working within the narrow confines of that paradigm has presented problems for childbirth educators and even obstetrical nurses, making it hazardous for them to become outspoken advocates for the fully sentient babies being repeatedly traumatized at birth.

In the era of industrialized medicine, the refined quality of both infant and maternal *awareness* has been clumsily overlooked and suppressed. What began with concern for mothers in labor pain now ends with *routine* use of multiple anesthetics and a cascade of other interferences—monitoring, drips, artificial rupture of membranes, artificial oxytocin, and dramatic surgical rescues in the form of Cesareans whether technically needed or not! All this mightily distracts mothers and babies from doing what they might otherwise accomplish more safely and proudly together, minus the psychic collateral damage.

Calm Birth raises urgent questions about the mental and emotional quality of birth today and offers well-tested methods to help mothers take more responsibility for themselves and their babies. The prospect of reducing complications while increasing maternal feelings of dignity and triumph should warm the hearts of all birth attendants.

As a psychologist, I rejoice in the idea of pregnancy as a Master Path for parents and look forward to the contributions of meditation science to an expanding vision of pregnancy and childbirth. Welcome, Calm Birth!

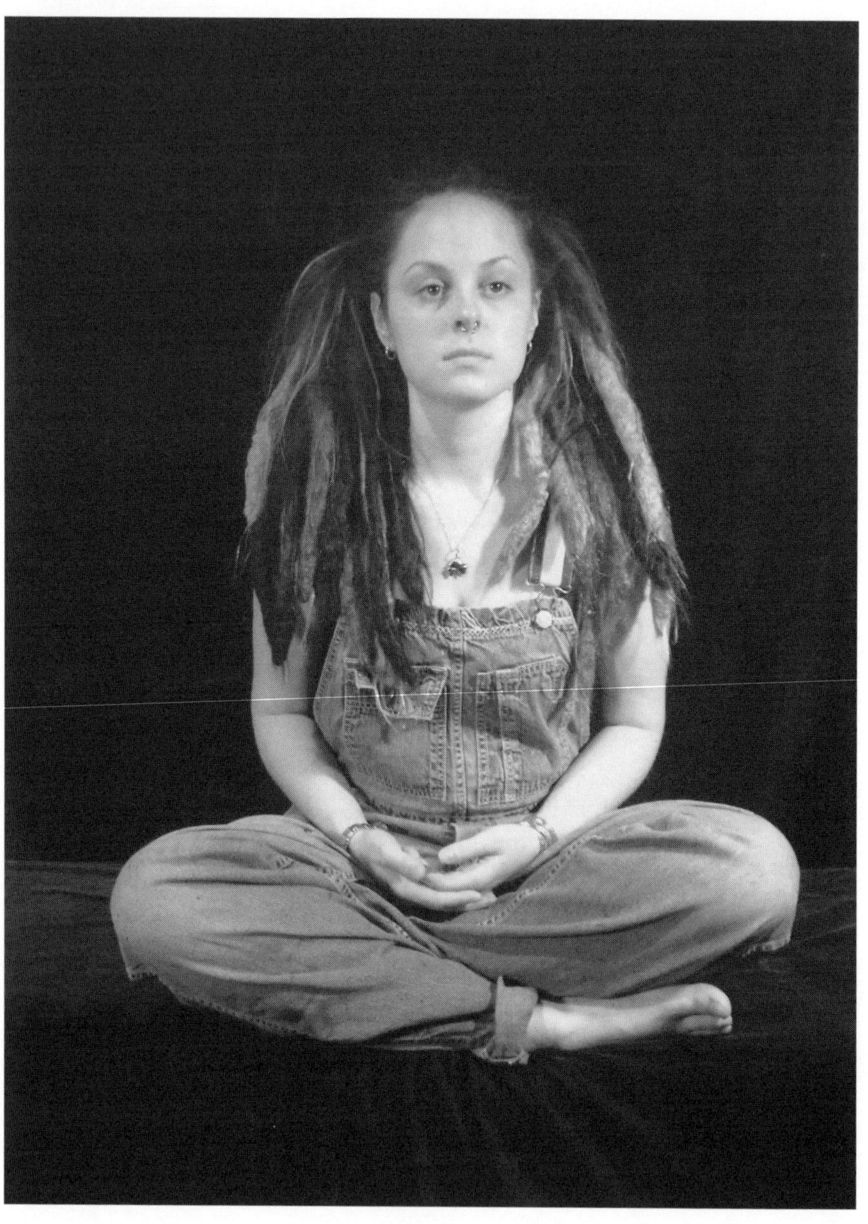

Preface

The opening up of a new paradigm is humbling and exhilarating; we were not so much wrong as partial, as if we had been seeing with a single eye. It is not more knowledge but a new knowing.

—Marilyn Ferguson, *The Aquarian Conspiracy*

THE SHIFT IN THE MEDICAL PARADIGM is multidimensional. It lets us see with new eyes how deeply we need new childbirth methods. It lets us see that what we need is now possible. It lets us know how new childbirth methods may be a factor in evolution.

Marsden Wagner, Ph.D., a scientist who has done important research for the World Health Organization on the extensive use of medical interventions in childbirth, has reported that the frequent use of inadequately evaluated medical interventions risks adverse health consequences and has escalated health care costs (Wagner, 1994). Decades of malpractice lawsuits have been driving up the cost of childbirth and have been driving doctors out of obstetrics. The lawsuits, persistent problems of low birth weight and premature birth, Cesarean deliveries at 26 percent and rising, and the unbearable costs of neonatal intensive care are signs of failure in maternal-infant care in the U.S. health care system.

The medical insurers have made it very difficult for women to give birth at home even though home births are at least as safe as hospital births, and avoid the risks that come with the medical interventions prevalent in the hospitals. Primarily due to medical insurance regulations, currently about 99 percent of childbirths take place in hospitals, which have had a stifling effect on natural birth. Even highly motivated women who have prepared earnestly for natural childbirth have been overpowered in the hospital environment. The Lamaze program, the most popular natural childbirth program from the 1950s onward in the USA and Europe, currently has epidural anesthesia rates of more than 70 percent. As Dr. Chamberlain discloses in his foreword to this book, cultural factors and insurance regulations have effectively channeled women into hospital birth—a relatively new form of birthing (unnatural birth) which hasn't proved to be safe or right. Despite strong national trends in the direction of alternative types of health care, in the important field of maternal-infant care, where alternatives to medical birth are needed, the Dick-Read, Lamaze, and Bradley programs have little impact today as normal birth alternatives.

Emerging Possibilities

To many childbirth professionals the situation seems dark. Are there any factors that may bring light into the field of childbirth science? The answer is definitely YES.

The world constantly changes, and medical science has been changing in ways that clearly encourage new directions for childbirth methodology. Between 1993 and 1996 three important educators described changes in the medical paradigm vital for the sake of national health and welfare.

Larry Dossey, M.D., a widely respected medical doctor with a brilliant ability to elucidate the history and progress of medical science, published his description of "the Three Eras of Medicine" in 1993. In his book *Healing Words,* the first of his books to become best sellers, he brought widespread attention to the development and potential of new health care methodology. Dossey's books, and other important publications of mind/body medicine, were one of the factors effecting popular demand for an increase in availability of mind/body methods, a demand that influenced both medical and nursing schools to include alternative methods in their curriculums.

In brief, Dr. Dossey describes Era One Medicine as the scientific (deterministic, or materialistic) medicine that began developing in the late 19th century and flourished during and after World War II. This is still the prevailing methodology today, intent on diagnosing, suppressing, or surgically removing physical symptoms. Era Two Medicine emerged in America in the late 1960s and the 1970s with a significant interest at Harvard, and then at the University of Massachusetts Medical Center (UMMC), in the importance of mind/body methods such as meditation. These interventions proved to have remarkable biological benefits, especially with respect to stress and anxiety, which have been increasingly associated with disease development. A factor in the development of Era Two mind/body methodology has been the increasing presence of meditation science traditions in the West, offering authoritative presentations of methods refined through centuries of use and supported by revered literature, increasingly available in English translation. The body of contemporary research that has developed studying the application of mind/body methods, and meditation methods in particular, is now renowned. More than fifteen thousand research papers and books have been published on the effects of this methodology in recent years.

Era Three Medicine is described by Dr. Dossey as "transpersonal." It is universal field medicine (see Chapter V, *Giving and Receiving*), including such interventions as intercessory prayer and long-distance healing, now supported by a growing body of research.

A second luminary of changes in the medical paradigm is Herbert Benson, M.D., the Harvard Medical School cardiologist who was an important early leader in the research and publications concerning meditation. Following the renowned work of Dr. Hans Selye in the 1950s on the biology of stress, a growing concern in the era of the Cold War, Benson brought widespread attention to meditation, an intervention of great potential importance as an antidote to stress and anxiety. In 1996 he published his book *Timeless Healing*, based on more than thirty years of research and clinical experience in mind/body medicine at Harvard. In the book he describes the most essential intervention for the emerging medical paradigm as self-care, the most proven methods of which are mind/body practices, particularly meditation. With self-care at the heart of a revolutionized health care system, said Dr. Benson, drugs and surgery would be used less and used more appropriately. Health care costs would decline and the standards and quality of our health care system would improve.

A third important description of a needed and available change in health care was published by Norman Shealy, M.D., Ph.D., and Carolyn Myss, Ph.D., in *The Creation of Health* (1993). Myss articulated the needed revolution in health care to be a shift of power from doctor to patient. In the medical system that still prevails, the doctor is most often too powerful and keeps the patient in a position of weakness, which is not good for the patient's health. In a transfer of power to the patient as the primary healer, patients would be empowered with information and methods enabling them to take a vital role in their own health and healing, with self-care methods being of central importance, and education in the use of those methods being essential.

Childbirth science could be making significant use of the self-empowering mind/body methods now available. They are in the public domain and are known to medical science. The application of mind/body medicine and meditation science to prenatal care could raise the quality and standards of childbirth health care. The public must be helped to understand that important methods are available that can bring childbirth science into a new era. Obstetrics is the area of medicine that has been most resistant to new methodologies of the expanded medical paradigm, methods that may have their most important application in childbirth.

Meditation is most often empowering. With proper instruction and use it has important health results for most people. The large majority of people who practice meditation properly have experienced significant biological and psychological improvements. Among the various complementary and alternative medicines (CAM) that have drawn so much interest internationally, meditation is the most proven. Meditation is an established complement to allopathic medicine and is important to the advance of medical science today. Research has demonstrated that meditation is clinically effective in both short- and long-term applications. More than eighteen thousand people, including many medical professionals, have trained in the mindfulness meditation techniques offered at the UMMC. Meditation's proven benefits of hormonal balancing, immune system enhancement, symptom reduction, and pain management are documented by major studies. The potential of childbirth meditation is great.

Development of Calm Birth

When I was young I wanted to be a doctor. I enrolled in college and studied in a pre-med program. Then I switched majors and received a BA degree from the University of California at Berkeley in science and communications. It was after college that my real studies began. In 1967 I began to work with teachers trained in profound methods from meditation science traditions. In 1970 I began a ten-year study and practice of *shamatha-vipashyana*[1] meditation with Chögyam Trungpa Rinpoche, a Vajrayana[2] Buddhist meditation master. This practice is essentially the same one used by Dr. Jon Kabat-Zinn in the UMMC medicine/meditation program. From 1980 to the present, I have been working with *Vajrayana* meditation masters who are also doctors. I was trained for many years in a deep breathing method called *Vase Breathing,* which became the

1. See glossary.
2. *Vajrayana* (Tibetan Buddhism), the "Diamond Vehicle," meditation science tradition.

basis of my work in the medical uses of meditation. The method has extraordinary potential for application to childbirth.

Though I've taught various courses in colleges and universities, my teaching of meditation remained private until 1991. It was then, with Drs. John Sutton and Craig Spaniol of NASA, that we incorporated MediGrace, Inc. for the research and development of methods of energy medicine and mind/body science. The first MediGrace program developed was Medical Uses of Meditation, a medicine/meditation program using three methods: the *Practice of Self-Care; Vase Breathing;* and *Reversal of Suffering*. From 1997 through 2004, more than sixty Medical Uses of Meditation trainings were presented in West Coast hospitals, with education credits granted by the California Board of Nursing. The second program that evolved was Calm Birth, a program of new childbirth methods. A Calm Birth pilot program was presented in Southern Oregon hospitals in 1998 and 1999. From its inception the program has involved the work of many medical and childbirth professionals. It has received grants from the Rockefeller Foundation and the Health Research Institute. Currently the program is available up and down the West Coast, from Southern California to Seattle.

Calm Birth can be considered an extension of the work of Grantly Dick-Read (*Childbirth without Fear,* 1944) and Robert Bradley (*Husband-Coached Childbirth,* 1965). Dick-Read's work didn't have the cultural availability of sophisticated psychological meditation methods now able to expose and release fear in childbirth (see Chapter V, *Womb Breathing*). Bradley's work didn't have methods available that would enable a man to directly bond with the awareness of the womb child, with developmental potential, and to bond with his wife in her practice of prenatal healing. Such methods are now available (see Chapter V). The Calm Birth method is not the "Newman Method" because it is history that has made methods of a higher order available. As Victor Hugo said, "Genius is an idea whose time has come." I have decades of training in the methods, and that allows me to teach them correctly.

Overview of the Program

THERE ARE THREE MAIN METHODS in the Calm Birth program: *Practice of Opening*, *Womb Breathing*, and *Giving and Receiving*, and the program also teaches instinctive and sacred movement. *Practice of Opening* is a progressive relaxation method, with healing neuromuscular release, based on mind/body science. It allows the pregnant woman and her partner to experience a remarkable access to the development of the unborn child. *Womb Breathing* is based on the *Vase Breathing* meditation method taught by Tibetan *Vajrayana* masters. This practice offers a new vision of the body and potential of the pregnant woman. With *Womb Breathing* women learn to breathe into their energy body to reach full potential in childbirth, to profoundly enrich the child. This practice extends natural labor pain management. The third method, *Giving and Receiving*, is a treasure from ancient wisdom used to bring healing into childbirth. Variants of all three of these methods have been developed for women to use in postnatal care. In prenatal care the program facilitates instinctive movement for optimal capability; for postnatal care the program teaches sacred movement for empowerment. The postnatal movements are from the Magical Passes of the Toltec lineage, as revealed by Carlos Castaneda, and from sacred temple dance.

When pregnant women practice meditation an empowering sense of safety and wholeness is generated from the inside. The Calm Birth methods were developed to give women direct ways to raise the quality of health in childbirth, whether or not medical interventions are applied. Calm Birth is complementary medicine; it can be very beneficial if drugs, anesthesia, and surgery are used. It strengthens the immune system and helps women and infants manage the side effects of medical interventions. It strengthens women psychologically and reduces the impact of birth-related shock and trauma. Calm Birth lowers medical costs and risks. It's most beneficial when used as primary care.

Given the controversial status of obstetrical practices today, and given the widespread interest in alternative health care, let us strongly consider the application of methods of benign mind/body science in childbirth. The availability of such methods is an important chance to raise the quality of health in the basis of life.

—Robert Bruce Newman, April 2005

I

Background

Women have always been healers. Cultural myths from around the world describe a time when only women knew the secrets of life and death, and therefore they alone could practice the magical art of healing.... The emergence of women whose consciousness blends with the ancient themes of healing is the single most promising event in health care....

—Jeanne Achterberg, *Woman as Healer*

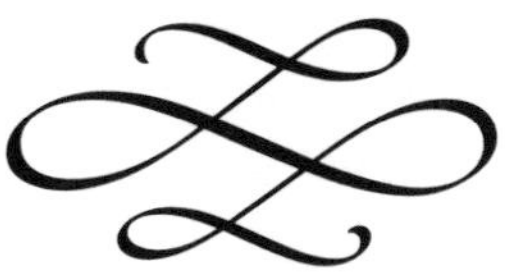

Repression of the Natural Genius of Women

In 1998 I read Jeanne Achterberg's highly respected book, *Imagery in Healing* (1985), a well-researched classic of mind/body medicine. In it is a concise chapter called "Imagery and the History of Medicine." I read it and was as shocked as I've ever been. I wept, both for empathetically realizing what happened in a terrible period of Western history and for not having known.

> In the midst of the atmosphere of change brought about by the issuance of the official mandates determining who should administer to the sick ... one of the saddest events in the history of women and healing began: the great witch hunt. It was inordinately successful in eliminating women's influence on the healing arts up to the present day. In fact, it was inordinately successful in eliminating women, period. Estimates are that anywhere from a few hundred thousand to nine million women were murdered between the years 1500 and 1650, many of them for the suspicioned practice of medicine (Achterberg, 1985, p. 67).

I considered myself a well-educated, well-informed person, but I was ignorant about how many women were tortured and murdered in "Renaissance" Europe, and then in America, often for practicing healing arts or midwifery. Following is what my further research found.

Throughout the centuries of history, childbirth took place among women. Childbirth everywhere was in the hands of skilled midwives and other women, family and friends. There were women of wisdom who were called upon as needed. Spiritual knowledge of childbirth[3] was transmitted through the ages in the Wise Woman

3. In today's childbirth we are missing great knowledge from the Wise

tradition. Childbirth was in the right hands.

Then, in the 16th and 17th centuries, came the Church of the Inquisition and the widespread execution of women of the families of Europe. It was the ultimate witch hunt, through more than two centuries. Women who practiced healing arts and midwifery were primary targets. Women traditionally had not only the responsibility and knowledge to take care of childbirth; they also had profound and widely respected medicine traditions, and they took care of the dying. But Europe was ravaged and impoverished by war and disease coming out of the Middle Ages into the "Renaissance." The competition for resources was severe. Only men were allowed to study medicine. If a woman showed a gift for healing, she was usually damned by the Church as having obtained power through alliance with the devil; to male doctors it usually meant that she was practicing medicine without a license, something they controlled.

And so it proceeded that for more than two hundred years, with twisted Church authorities suspecting women in general of readiness for pacts with the devil, that the persecution, torture, and murder of women devastated Europe and then America. Some men were perfect accomplices, especially doctors and other professionals organizing to protect their authority. They gave backbone and fire to the holocaust. Burning was the favored means of murder. Alliance of Church and state conspired to create "the shocking nightmare, the foulest crime, and deepest sense of shame of Western civilization, the blackout of everything that Homo sapiens, the reasoning man, has ever upheld" (Achterberg, 1990, p. 88).

The institutionalization of the trials, tortures, and executions was well documented. It was the lowest level of aggressive, competitive greed in nations short of money and weak in industry, based

---

Women era. When the Wise Woman tradition was destroyed important knowledge was lost. Now we can see that perhaps it's been waiting to be rediscovered.

on the power of the Church to accuse and to sanction killing. Man against woman. "The charge of witchcraft became the single most effective means of controlling the monopoly of the healing professions" (ibid., p. 83). "Midwifery and folk healing—risky occupations in which the practitioner was doubly damned—were alternatives to starvation" (ibid., p. 88). Sometimes women were allowed to practice midwifery, but the profession had a bad reputation and was dangerous. Midwives were often fined, imprisoned, or killed if the outcome of their work was considered a failure, that is, a stillborn or deformed child.

Reemergence of Medicine Women

THE TERM *Homo sapiens* means wisdom man and wisdom woman. In a dark period of Western civilization, the natural gifts of the wisdom woman were repressed with torture and murder. Woman's work as a healer and her use of important knowledge of childbirth, vital resources of the West, were almost obliterated. But the species silently survived. Male doctors continued to organize and professionalize their business, taking over childbirth.

Coming into the 18th century, the persecution of woman the healer and midwife slowly stopped. But for centuries after the destruction of the Wise Woman tradition, natural childbirth options were generally not available for women due to possible prosecution. Licensed doctors, always men, were most often called upon to deliver children.

Coming into the 20th century, obstetrics and gynecology were predominantly male professions in which the interventions of medical science were being applied more and more, forming a tradition of unnatural childbirth. Today there are increasing numbers of women OB/GYNs in our medical system, but women, in general, in our culture are still not instructed about natural birth options.

Natural childbirth programs began to develop in the West in the

20th century by way of two European doctors, Grantly Dick-Read of England and Fernand Lamaze of France. They both stirred interest in normal childbirth in Europe and America. Late in the 20th century, when it was clear that the quality of human health was at risk from the uncontrolled use of anesthesia, surgery, and strong drugs in childbirth, the natural childbirth programs of Dick-Read, Lamaze, and Bradley drew the attention of many women. In those childbirth education programs women found that instruction in natural childbirth capability and prenatal care was essential for making conscious decisions affecting health in childbirth.

Toward the end of the 20th century, teachers from revered meditation traditions coming into the West became an increasing resource of wisdom and methods. This resource is now being brought into childbirth and is helping women discover remarkable innate capability and find healing in the childbirth process. These methods from ancient wisdom inspiring new natural childbirth methodology give women the option to make childbirth a process of personal realization and development, and at the same time protect the evolutionary potential of the species.

The Wise Woman tradition is emerging anew. One way it emerges is when it comes from within as women practice energy medicine and healing methods in preparation for childbirth, lifting themselves into their inherent wisdom.

New Childbirth Anatomy and Potential

It started late in the 20th century, and now early in the 21st century a force of history is expanding the vision of childbirth anatomy and the potential of normal birth.

In meditation science traditions available throughout the West, people learn to breathe energy for greater function. In *Zen* Buddhist meditation people breathe down into the *Hara*, the vital navel center, for optimal function. In *Vajrayana* Buddhist meditation people learn to breathe energy down into the Life Vase in the navel center, to send energy up the central energy channel. In *Tai Chi*, people sink *chi* into the *tan tien*, in the navel, for vital force and realization. Widespread interest in the work of Carlos Castaneda finds a Toltec tradition of great knowledge. In this native Western lineage, women are known to be able to see energy and to use their wombs to process knowledge directly for evolution. Something remarkable has become evident in America. Traditional wisdom knows how to breathe energy. Breathing energy into the energy body is a known human ability. The ability to breathe energy into the navel center in the energy body is an important human resource.

Now, as more and more women practice meditation, when they become pregnant and practice they're taking superior prenatal care. Some women practice breathing energy into the Life Vase in the energy body to benefit the birth. For such women pregnancy has become an empowering master path. If energy breathing meditation is applied as a primary prenatal care method, conception to delivery may progress as a path in which women empower themselves to avoid dangers of medical interventions and to bring illumination into childbirth. Women who use such methods are practicing energy medicine for childbirth.

II

Childbirth Meditation

Meditation is not just a practice, it is a way of life. Initially that way of life is learned through formal practice, just as we learn to play a musical instrument in this fashion. Some people will choose to continue practice periods and others won't, but both will have shifted the paradigm through which they relate to the world.

—Joan and Miroslav Borysenko, *The Power of the Mind to Heal*

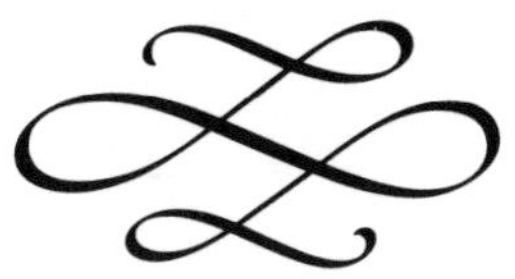

Introduction

Both the words *medicine* and *meditation* come from the Latin word *mederi,* which means "to cure." Medicine refers to methods for the curing of symptoms of disease. Meditation refers to methods that go deeper, to shift and improve human function. Meditation is a consciousness discipline that enables people to experience greater levels of awareness and intelligence and greater levels of health, normally blocked by the mind in its undisciplined activity. Meditation science is the basis of profound traditions and has extensive knowledge of short- and long-term benefits of proven methods. Contemporary science has defined meditation as having five main characteristics: specific method; muscle relaxation; logic relaxation (that is, to suspend analyzing, judging, and expectation); self-induced state; and control of attention (Cardoso et al., 2004, pp. 58–60). Childbirth meditation is the application of traditional meditation methods as enrichment practice in prenatal care and in postnatal care.

With the progressive increase of the presence of meditation lineages and traditionally trained meditation teachers in the West in the past fifty years, and with meditation now widely accepted as a valuable health enhancement factor, many thousands of women who practice meditation have experienced benefits during pregnancy and labor. Some women who have no experience of meditation seek meditation and yoga methods to benefit their pregnancies. Childbirth meditation is an important subject for research. It may impact childbirth medicine for a long time to come. Childbirth meditation may be the key to a needed revolution in childbirth science.

Advanced natural childbirth refers to childbirth methods in which new applications of meditation practices empower women to adhere to and advance the principles of natural childbirth. In this book we discuss specific advanced natural childbirth methods. In describing the method of *Womb Breathing,* we will discuss a new vision of childbirth anatomy that includes energy body anatomy.

The Increasing Presence of Meditation in the West

THE PRESENCE OF MEDITATION in Western life in the post Cold War era has become ubiquitous.

> Meditation ... is fast appearing in unexpected places throughout modern American culture. Secretaries are doing it as part of their daily noon yoga classes. Pre-adolescent teenagers dropped off at the YMCA by their mothers on a Saturday morning are learning it as part of their karate training. Truck drivers and housewives in the Stress Reduction Program at the University of Massachusetts Medical Center are practicing a combination of Hindu yoga and Buddhist insight meditation to control hypertension [and pain]. Star athletes prepare themselves for a demanding basketball game with centering techniques learned in Zen (Murphy and Donovan, 1999, p. 1).

The increasing use of meditation in all aspects of medicine has been remarkable. Since the start of the landmark research at the Harvard Medical School in the 1960s, and particularly since the advent of the medicine/meditation program at the University of Massachusetts Medical Center (UMMC) starting in 1979, meditation has been widely researched and used increasingly in medical applications. The comprehensive review compiled by Murphy and Donovan (1999) enables us to appraise the vast research on the benefits of meditation and to evaluate the benefits pertaining to childbirth.

Benefits of Childbirth Meditation

The following is a brief overview of the psychological and physiological benefits of meditation that may be imparted to a womb child through the pregnant woman's bloodstream and through sympathetic resonance. The same benefits, in general, may be imparted to the child after birth with postnatal meditation through lactation and breast-feeding and through sympathetic resonance. At all times childbirth meditation benefits are dual, inseparably benefiting the woman and the child. In addition, in a larger sense, meditation can be seen to be benefiting the family and society in general.

Biological Benefits of Meditation

This subject has become vast, but with respect to directly affecting the quality of childbirth, the focus will be primarily on three areas: hormonal balance, immune system enhancement, and pain management.

Our era has been called the age of anxiety. It's been well proven that anxiety and resultant stress are key factors in health, and are significant causes in most disease and adverse psychological conditions. As extensive research has shown, meditation is a noninvasive antidote to biological and psychological problems caused by anxiety and stress.

In brief, anxiety causes an overproduction of the hormones adrenaline and cortisol, which suppress important biological functions in order to shift energy into muscle systems for a "fight or flight" reaction, based on old instinctive tendencies. Anxiety suppresses immune system function primarily through elevated levels of cortisol in the bloodstream. Anxiety, with accompanying hormonal imbalance, has been proven, through extensive research, to be a primary factor in the weakening of health and the cause of various immune-deficiency diseases.

The widespread chemical treatment of anxiety has resulted in additional biological and psychological problems. If a woman is pregnant, the treatment of anxiety with mood-modulating chemicals can result in birth defects or other long-term health problems.

In contrast, self-calming meditation has been shown to directly reduce adrenaline and cortisol secretion, naturally restoring hormonal balance in general and normalizing immune system function. In addition meditation produces elevated levels of the major hormones melatonin, DHEA, and serotonin, and endorphins, powerful pain-relieving, pleasure-causing agents secreted by the nervous system.

Melatonin

The fact that meditation produces elevated levels of melatonin, the hormone secreted by the pineal gland located at the center of the brain, was first disclosed by research conducted at the University of Massachusetts Medical Center in 1995. The pineal gland has drawn the attention of human insight for a long time. In sacred literature more than twenty-five hundred years old, the Vedas of India described the pineal gland in the context of the energy body:

> The [pineal] gland was portrayed as one of the seven *chakras,* or centers of vital energy, which are arranged along the central axis of the body. The pineal gland was thought to be the supreme or crown chakra ... the ultimate center of spiritual force (Reiter and Robinson, 1995, p. 131).

In the 17th century, Descartes, in his famous *Treatise of Man,* called the pineal gland the seat of the human psyche, the principal location of self-awareness. The above insights are inspiring concerns for people interested in meditation.

Current worldwide interest in melatonin, evident in the presence of hundreds of research papers and books on the subject, is focused on its biological benefits, particularly concerning the remarkable effects of melatonin on the human immune system. Melatonin many be the most potent and versatile antioxidant. It directly stimulates interleukin-2 activity, which in turn stimulates the increase of all the various cells of the immune system, in a pervasive optimization of immune function. Melatonin directly restores and increases T-helper cell production in bone marrow.

In stress-inducing times, which tend to cause detrimental hormonal imbalances, strong levels of melatonin intentionally produced by pregnant women indicate that they are engaged in effective prenatal care. Melatonin is renowned as a sleep-aid. Especially when produced naturally to elevated levels, it assures normal sleep and rest even in challenging situations.

The practice of meditation has been proven to be superior to deep sleep in bringing about energy restoration and repair. Thus meditation offers a natural means of physiological and psychological refreshment vital for a healthy childbirth outcome. Melatonin is known to have a calming effect, bringing contentment and improved mood. In our times, a pregnant woman's self-induced meditation calm may be a womb child's greatest need; without it, the woman and child may be vulnerable to various interventions and disturbances.

To summarize, the natural production of elevated levels of melatonin in meditation, conveyed to the child prenatally through the woman's bloodstream and postnatally through breast-feeding, gives remarkable immune enhancement and overall health benefits. Though the extensive research in melatonin benefits has been concentrated almost entirely on the above, there are probable intelligence enhancement benefits for the child warranting research.

DHEA (dehydroepiandrosterone)

Increased levels of DHEA, a life-enhancing hormone, were one of the first biological benefits of meditation to be observed. DHEA is produced in the adrenal glands, just above the kidneys.

Like melatonin, DHEA has a variety of health-affecting benefits. It is an immunity enhancement agent that has been proven to be beneficial in the prevention and treatment of cancer, cardiovascular disease, diabetes, lupus, and other disorders. DHEA stimulates the production of monocytes (T cells and B cells), potent immunity biochemicals that cause the production of other immune system agents. T cells (white blood cells produced in the bone marrow) produce two powerful immune system agents: interleukin-2 and gamma-interferon, intelligent defense agents that help maintain health. DHEA is good for the bones, muscles, blood pressure, vision, and hearing. It is the substance from which the male and female hormones are developed. It contributes to vitality and youthfulness. DHEA is a mood elevator that makes people feel and look better. It enhances brain biochemistry and growth. Anxiety and stress lower normal DHEA levels in the bloodstream. Meditation elevates DHEA levels. Thus meditation during pregnancy, in offering potentially ideal hormonal function, generates elevated levels of vivifying DHEA in the woman's bloodstream, which benefits the womb child. If the mother keeps meditating after birth the child receives the DHEA enrichment through lactation and breast-feeding.

Serotonin

Another important hormone produced in elevated amounts in meditation, with important implications for childbirth, is serotonin. It is a natural substance the body uses to make melatonin. Serotonin is a neurotransmitter produced in the brain and in the guts ("inner and deeper parts") that has a calming effect, associated with contentment. It also regulates blood vessel elasticity, helps repair muscle tissue damage, and is generally beneficial in healing. It is conveyed from woman to child in the same way as melatonin and DHEA.

Endorphins

Meditation is also known to produce endorphins, peptides secreted throughout the nervous system that have a very strong pain-relieving and pleasure-inducing effect, similar to that of morphine. Deepak Chopra writes:

> Thus the brain [and nervous system in general] produces narcotics up to 200 times stronger than anything you can buy . . . with the added boon that our own pain-killers are non-addictive. Morphine and endorphins both block pain by filling a certain receptor on the neuron and preventing other chemicals that carry the message of pain from coming in, without which there can be no sensation of pain, no matter how much physical provocation is present (1990, p. 62).

Michel Odent observes that the longer and more challenging the labor, the higher the level of endorphins (1994, p. 15). With respect to childbirth meditation, it is probable that the more time that is devoted to the practice of prenatal meditation the higher the level of endorphins during labor and at birth. Thus women who meditate for childbirth probably have optimal endorphin levels supporting the potential of natural childbirth. This is a very important subject for research.

Endorphin production is important to a woman in avoiding the risks of medical interventions and in gaining confidence in her natural abilities in childbirth. Candace Pert (1997) writes about her third childbirth:

> ... my magic bullet had been breathing, which is a surefire, proven strategy for releasing endorphins and quelling pain. Obviously, this is what previous generations of women, in the days before IV drips and synthetic painkillers, had relied on. Both they and their babies must have been better off for the experience, as I certainly felt myself to be (p. 167).

Meditation and Pain Management

Another important benefit derived from meditation is increased tolerance of pain based on psychological factors. Extensive research conducted at the UMMC (Murphy and Donovan, 1999, pp. 77–78) demonstrated significant reductions in the following: present moment pain, negative body image, inhibition of activity (movement limitation), psychological disturbance, anxiety and depression, and the need for pain-related drugs.

With the mindfulness meditation method used at the UMMC, people learn to distinguish between mind and awareness. They are instructed to shift attention from mind to awareness and to experience a vital change of function. As people learn to expose mind to awareness, they learn to see how the mind dwells on anxiety and fear and burns up energy, exhausting them and limiting their ability. With mindfulness meditation they learn that they're capable of staying in the present moment, even while experiencing high levels of pain. They see that their mind likes to avoid being present by making a big deal about the pain. They see that for deep reasons they want to stay in open awareness and avoid mind.

People practicing mindfulness meditation see that they can develop fearlessness and gain energy by staying with pain sensations, avoiding letting their mind agonize and waste energy reserves. They see that they have a choice to prevent distress and build courage and inner strength in the process.

These results point out how meditation has important potential application in labor pain management, both to avoid unnecessary anguish and to avoid the use of risky medical interventions (see Chapter V, *Womb Breathing*). Staying with present moment pain naturally releases endorphins, increasing the ability to stay present. The more one is willing to face the pain, the higher the endorphin levels and the greater the development of fearlessness.

Psychological Benefits of Meditation

Murphy and Donovan (1999) describe extensive research in the following psychological benefits of meditation:

- Reaction Time and Physical Motor Skill
- Field Independence
- Concentration and Intelligence
- Empathy
- Creativity
- Self-Actualization

It is observed, in brief, that various meditation schools offer methods to cultivate clarity, flexibility, efficiency, and a broadened range of functions. This is seen in the meditation results reviewed in the fifty-one pages of research abstracts in the Murphy and Donovan book (p. 81ff).

The above cognitive benefits produced by meditation in a pregnant woman entrain the womb child to develop vital cognitive qualities. Hopefully future research will seek to observe and compare traits developed in children exposed to childbirth meditation with traits developed in children without that exposure.

Research Directions

Observed benefits of meditation with significant implications for childbirth are as follows: Benson (1996) noted Cesarean section surgery reduced by 56 percent and epidural anesthesia use reduced by 85 percent among meditators; Astin et al. (1987) concluded that mindfulness meditation may be an important coping strategy for transforming the ways in which we respond to life events.

Altogether, increased pain management skills and increased levels of endorphins, serotonin, and other hormones, all attributable to meditation, should be important incentives for women who don't want to risk chemicals and anesthesia in childbirth.

A pregnant woman's meditation always has dual benefits. The woman communicates psychologically and energetically, influencing the child to produce healthful neurohormones and neurotransmitters. And she communicates hormonal benefits through her bloodstream to the child. If anesthesia is used, and/or drugs, some of which are toxic (Davis-Floyd, 2003, p. 99), childbirth meditation may importantly counter side effects of the medicine in them both. This is an essential subject for research (see pp. 220–22).

Discovering More Dimensions of Life

As we discover more and more dimensions of physiological and psychological function, and as meditation science becomes more valuable to childbirth medicine and more the focus of research in childbirth science, we'll learn more about the potential of meditation in childbirth. Looking into the field of that potential, we can see two great forces. One is the inevitable use of energy medicine in childbirth; the other is the inherent potential for childbirth to become a master path.

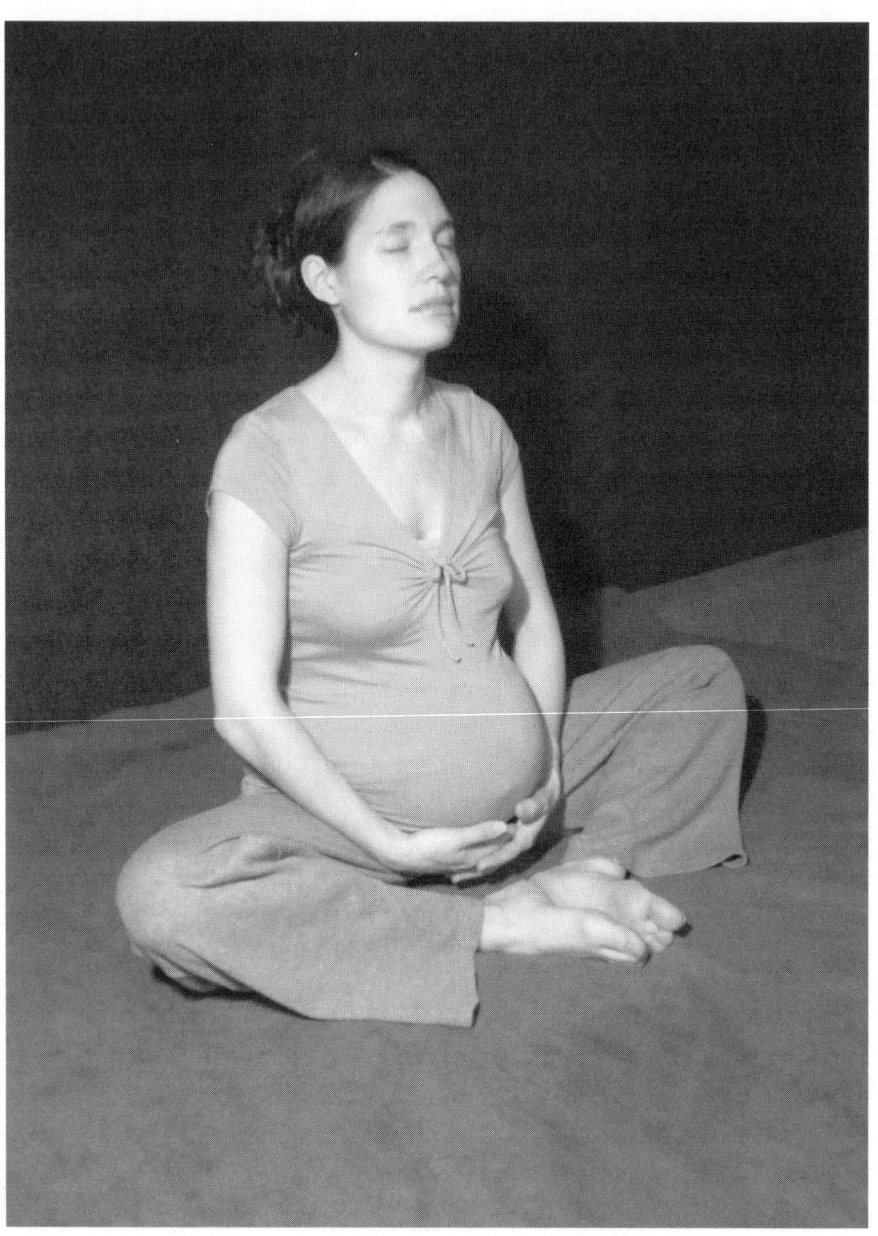

III

Childbirth and Energy Medicine

. . . intuitive or symbolic sight is not a gift but a skill—a skill based in self-esteem. Developing this skill—and a healthy sense of self—becomes easier when you can think in the words, concepts and principles of energy medicine.

—Caroline Myss, *Anatomy of the Spirit*

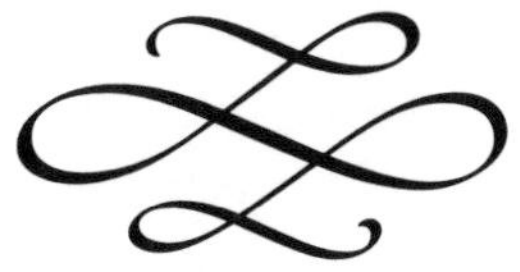

Transformed by the Energy of the Womb Child

FREDERICK LEBOYER'S SENSIBILITY penetrates to deep communion with the child in the womb. In his book *Birth without Violence* (1975),[4] he observed the potential of the meditative state in childbirth without having access to a method. The child becomes the teacher. Sensing what he calls the slowness of the time of the unborn child, Leboyer comments:

> Near-darkness ... silence ...
>
> A profound peace steals over everything, almost unnoticed.
>
> People don't raise their voices in church.
>
> On the contrary, instinctively, they lower them.
>
> And this too is a sacred place.
>
> Darkness and quiet, what more is needed?
>
> Patience.
>
> Or more accurately, the learning of an extreme slowness that comes close to immobility.
>
> Without acceptance of this slowness, success is impossible; without it, we cannot truly communicate with an infant.
>
> Relaxing, accepting the slow pace, letting it take command—all this requires training.
>
> As much for the mother as for those of us who attend her ...
>
> Without experiencing this extreme slowness in our own bodies, it is impossible to understand birth.
>
> Impossible to receive the newborn baby properly.
>
> His "time" is so slow as to approximate no movement at all.
>
> Ours is an agitation bordering on frenzy.
>
> Besides, we are never truly "here"—always "elsewhere."

4. Leboyer's book was published in French in 1974; Alfred A. Knopf, Inc. published the first edition in English in 1975.

In the past, with our memories; in the future, with our plans. Always "before" or "after." Never *now.*

But we must learn to be "here."

To forget the future, to forget the past.

Once again, everything is very simple.

And yet so hard to achieve.

How is it to be accomplished?

Only with the most passionate attention.

(1975, pp. 42–43)

In that book, Leboyer does not present a method. His writing is the expression of a gifted sensibility. The slowness, mindfulness of presence, and passionate attention are all qualities that have been available for centuries through traditional meditation training and practice.

In 1978 Leboyer published *Inner Beauty, Inner Light: Yoga for Pregnant Women.* He began with a loud WARNING about the dangers of this traditional method when used in pregnancy. He warned of the initial pain it will bring with every *asana,* every yogic posture. Yet he obviously felt the deep potential value of the discipline of yoga for prenatal care, with the right teacher. Again and again he emphasizes the need for a right teacher in yogic discipline, especially in prenatal care. He saw yoga as a method to master pain and fear that arise in childbirth. What was not in his experience was the safe method of sitting meditation, *dhyana asana,* as a central method, a complete method more gentle and safe than yoga, which is physically more forceful. It's true that sitting meditation as well as yogic postures is best practiced with the guidance of a teacher. But with the proper instruction sitting meditation can profoundly help a woman face fear and pain in childbirth, helping her to rely more on an inner teacher than an external teacher. Instruction for the psychological method of sitting meditation using energy breathing, physically relaxed compared to yoga, is becoming more generally available for women to use in childbirth. In energy body sitting meditation women learn a psychological method to work with fear and pain. Such energy body meditation methods, as developed in *Tai Chi, Qi Gong,* and *Vajrayana* Buddhist meditation, offer women a gentle approach to mastery and inner medicine.

Today such meditation methods offer women ways to slow down into their basic nature of intuitive wisdom, to patiently find more and more innate capability in childbirth. Prenatal meditation can be a great method for bonding, encouraging the woman to go inside, to slow down into the child, to be one with the energy of the child and its silent needs in coming to birth. Methods that unify the energy of the woman and the energy of the womb child bring energy medicine into birth.

Medicine Women Arising

IN 1974, THE YEAR of the publication of Leboyer's book in French, a twenty-five-year-old woman and mother of three published a book about the potential of natural childbirth and the importance of meditative discipline: *Prenatal Yoga and Natural Childbirth.* Jeannine Parvati Baker's language is superb and she shows us pregnancy as a master path, loaded with illumination potential. She learned *Zen* Buddhist meditation when she was a teenager, and later practiced both Buddhist and Hindu meditation methods. Jeannine developed a connection with energy breathing, which she used in her own births. Following are excerpts from her book:

> Giving birth is initiation into women's mysteries.... It prepares us for other altered states and dying to the self. Giving conscious birth is a woman's vision quest, par excellence.... Opening for conscious birth helps all power centers to open (Baker, 1974, p. xii).

> With breath as an ally we can receive a vision that will spiritually feed us our entire lives, right at the moment of conception and birth (p. xiii).

> ... new and powerful feelings and levels of consciousness brought about by being pregnant (p. 1).
>
> Women talk of their childbirth experiences being transcendent, mystical, and/or the most profound spiritual experiences of their lives (p. 18).
>
> Discipline is very much needed during pregnancy, not only from the ritual aspect, but to prepare for the great discipline required in caring for a baby (p. 2).
>
> [Referring to yoga teacher Hari Dass] I thanked him for the advice to concentrate on my navel *chakra* during labor as this transformed labor pains into the gifts they really are (p. 77).
>
> At the White Hole dimension of awareness, the personal dissolved—boundaries of self/other poured inside out with each birthforce wave. "Contractions" or labor pains were transformed into "gifts." Balancing between pleasure and pain brought power—power to be wisely used for the work at hand (p. 88).
>
> Tremendous release when the baby emerges—like pulling the universe through the eye of a needle (p. 90).
>
> ... and as the original definition of obstetrics is to "stand by," we can move out of the small space of fear (p. 101).

Jeannine Parvati Baker's natural childbirths included a spontaneous use of energy breathing. In Jeannine's own words she was "channeling from the earth how to integrate childbirth and meditation." Women have always instinctively used their breathing in childbirth. There is often a wisdom that arises in labor, guiding women to move and breathe in certain ways. In the last stages of the 20th century the medical establishment became interested in meditation and mind/body medicine, and that has encouraged the application of energy meditation in childbirth. Through meditation techniques now widely available, more and more women find that meditation helps them access instinctive wisdom, so that it arises more by method than by chance. They experience something of what Jeannine experienced. Her gifted use of language made her one of the first to lead the way to the use of meditation as energy medicine in childbirth.

The Use of Breath Meditation in Medicine

THE USE OF MIND/BODY METHODS in childbirth in the 20th century can be said to have begun with the work of Dick-Read and Lamaze. The use of energy medicine in childbirth is emerging. It includes and advances mind/body science.

For medicine in general, Dean Ornish made an important use of yogic breathing in his renowned heart care program.

> In this system, we inhale not only oxygen but also energy, or *prana*. In Sanskrit, *prana* means both breath and spirit ... breath is the vehicle for *prana*,... These techniques ... can expand the availability of energy to you (Ornish, 1990, p. 165).

Dr. Ornish recommends abdominal breathing as optimal for oxygenation and for energy:

> Breathing into your belly will gradually become automatic if you practice it on a regular basis. After a while you will breathe from your abdomen most of the time, even when you are asleep (p. 166).

In the Calm Birth program women learn how to practice *Womb Breathing* in their sleep, to breathe in a more profound and vital way. Demonstrations of the value of yogic breathing in medicine and childbirth and the growing interest in energy medicine make it inevitable and necessary to take methods that were used inside spiritual traditions and offer them to women to energize childbirth in ways that were not previously possible.

Universal Energy Medicine

IN THE SCIENCE OF YOGA, people inhale oxygen and subtle matter known as *prana,* or *chi,* or energy of the universal field. The human body is seen to have both physical and psychic energy channels. We're made to breathe both oxygen and energies of the universal field. Barbara Ann Brennan, a former NASA research scientist, has studied the characteristics of the universal energy field (UEF). In her book *Hands of Light* she describes the UEF comprehensively:

> The UEF has been known and observed throughout the ages. It has been studied as far back in history as we are able to reach. Each culture had a different name for the energy field phenomenon and looked at it from its particular viewpoint. When describing what it saw, each culture found similar basic properties in the UEF. As time progressed and the scientific method was developed, western culture began to investigate the UEF more rigorously. As the state of the art of our scientific equipment becomes more sophisticated, we are able to measure finer qualities of the UEF. From these investigations we can surmise that the UEF is probably composed of an energy previously undefined by western science, or possibly a matter of a finer substance than we generally considered matter to be. If we define matter as condensed energy, the UEF may exist between the presently considered realm of matter and that of energy. As we have seen, some scientists refer to the phenomenon of the UEF as bio-plasma[5] (Brennan, 1988, pp. 39–40).

5. *Bio-plasma* means protoplasm, the essential living matter of all plant and animal cells.

Revered traditions tell us that there is energy matter in the air that may be absorbed into human function. Whether we call it *prana*, or vital energies of the universal field, the question is: how do we absorb this energy and use it for greater function? Yogic science states that this energy absorption is well within human capability through the practice of specific breathing techniques refined through millenniums. The same energy absorption capability can be utilized in advanced childbirth methods. Its use in childbirth health care may be called an important application of energy medicine because of its potential significance to maternal-infant health.

Energy Medicine, Subtle and Powerful

James Oschman studies human energetic systems in his book, *Energy Medicine*, where he has concluded:

> Much of the seeming magic and mystery surrounding vibrational medicines is being revealed as the same mystery that has always been associated with the invisible yet palpable forces of nature. Many of the subtleties arising in the clinical context are none other than the subtleties of human structure and patterns of energy in interaction. As new research reveals the basis for these subtleties, we obtain a much clearer picture of the human body in health and disease. The medical and chemical-pharmacological models that have served us well in the past are not being replaced, but are being viewed within a more complete multidimensional perspective. "Subtle energies" and "dynamic energy systems" are neither supernatural nor do they require a revision of physics. They go to the foundation of life. The molecules and energy fields in our environment can affect living systems. An understanding of these relationships, whether based on intuition or on science, is fundamental to a wide range of therapeutic approaches … (Oschman, 2000, p. 145).

In the depths of a woman's natural sensitivity to internal and external energies, she has the inherent ability to breathe vital energies of the universal field into her systems. When she's pregnant she can access remarkable nourishment and awareness for the child by breathing energy. In doing so she can bring a new form of body and potential into childbirth, and she can help raise the paradigm of childbirth methodology for the sake of everyone.

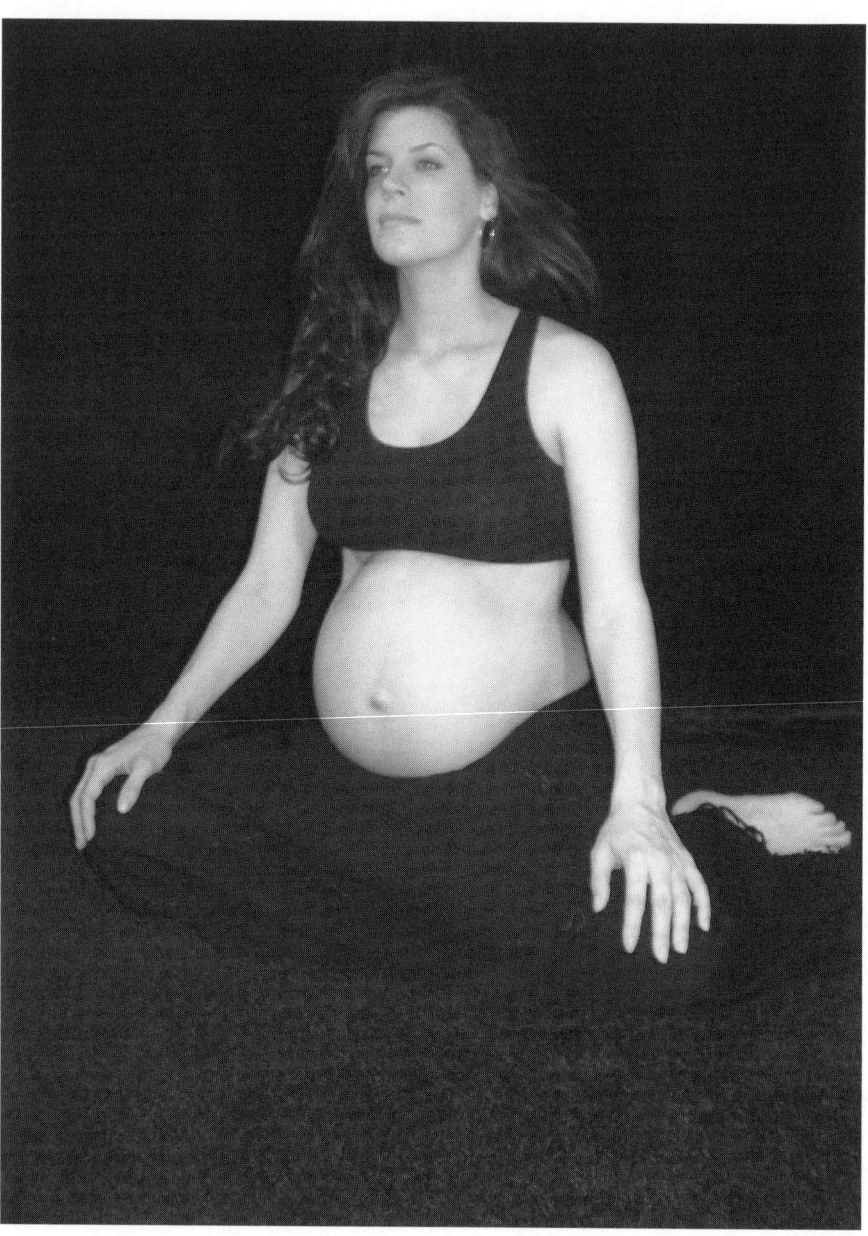

IV

Pregnancy as Master Path

Now we've all heard of yogis of the East and practitioners of certain mystical disciplines who have been able, through breath training, to alter their perception of physical pain. (Other people, known as mothers, demonstrate mastery equal to that of the yogis, when with proper training ... they use breathing techniques to control pain in childbirth).

—Candace Pert, *Molecules of Emotion*

The Liberation of the Womb

The Navel Center as a Natural Focus of Meditation

Hara, the Vital Center

Feeding Elixir into the Womb Child

Secret Instructions

The Life Vase and the Womb

Pain-Body Release

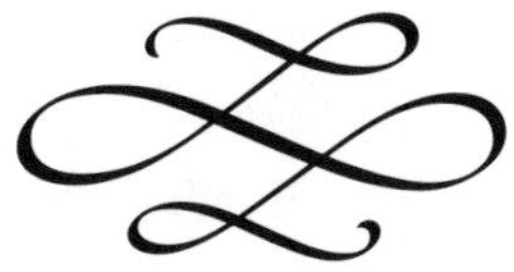

The Liberation of the Womb

THE WORK OF CARLOS CASTANEDA is important. It makes Western ancient wisdom available in our times. His unparalleled series of books on the Toltec lineage of Mexico brings to life teachers and teachings that are remarkably universal and valid for us today:

> According to don Juan Matus, one of the most specific interests of the shamans who lived in Mexico in ancient times was what they called the "liberation of the womb." He explained that the liberation of the womb entailed the awakening of its secondary functions, and that since the primary function of the womb, under normal circumstances, was reproduction, [they] were solely concerned with what they considered to be its secondary function: evolution. Evolution, in the case of the womb, was, for them, the awakening and full [use] of the womb's capacity to process direct knowledge.... Females can see energy directly more readily than males because of the effect of their wombs.... Women, because they have a womb, are so versatile, so individualistic in their ability to see energy directly that this accomplishment, which should be a triumph of the human spirit, is taken for granted (Castaneda, 1998, p. 71).

There are several truths here giving further meaning to what has been called the natural superiority of women (Montagu, 1954). Women have an inherent capacity to see energy. This is an extraordinary advantage in meditation practices in which vital essences in the air are sensed and breathed into the navel region, for storage and greater function, for realization and liberation.

The second significant advantage for the woman in traditional meditation practices that focus on breathing into the lower abdomen, shifting consciousness down and in, is that the womb can "process direct knowledge." Though Don Juan implies that women cannot use the womb for reproductive and evolutionary functions at the same time, with *Womb Breathing* women can use their reproductive function for the sake of evolution.

The Navel Center as a Natural Focus of Meditation

DR. CHENG MAN CH'ING shares secrets of his *Tai Chi* lineage, presenting the teachings as a martial art, as exercise, as medicine, and as a means of self-development. In his book, *Cheng Tzu's Thirteen Treatises on T'ai Chi Ch'uan* (1985) he states that beginners who start to learn *Tai Chi Chuan* should secure their mind and *chi*[6] in the *tan tien*. They must "sink the *chi* into the *tan tien*." In the book *chi* is sometimes translated as "breath." The *tan tien* is an energy body feature. The center of the *tan tien* is located behind the umbilicus, closer to the navel than the spine.

"When sinking the *chi* into the *tan tien*, the breathing must be fine, long, quiet and slow. Gradually inhale into the *tan tien* [breathing into the energy body]. The *chi* stays with the [awareness]. Then day after day, and month after month, the *chi* accumulates, naturally, without being forced" (p. 77). This accumulated *chi* is power for living more completely.

To develop *chi* naturally, as Lao-tzu explained, it is much like becoming as supple as an infant, flexible and receptive (p. 32). This is a good practice for pregnancy though it hasn't been intended as such. Focusing *chi* into the *tan tien* is focusing life force toward the womb. "Sinking the *chi* into the *tan tien* can give each internal organ

6. "*Chi [Qi]* is fundamental to Chinese medical thinking, yet no one English word or phrase can adequately capture its meaning. Perhaps we can think of *Qi* as matter on the verge of becoming energy or energy at the point of materializing" (Kaptchuk, 1983, p. 35).

its own exercise and stimulation for proper function" (p. 77).

Both for organ health and greater function, *Tai Chi* is excellent for prenatal care, offering an expanded vision of body and capability.

Hara, the Vital Center

ZEN MEDITATION IN JAPAN, transmitted from the Ch'an lineage of China, also features breathing into the navel center. The method is defined and explored in Karlfried Graf Von Durckheim's book *Hara* (1977). The *Hara*, "the honored middle," known as the primal center, contains the *tanden*, a focal point for meditation located two inches below the navel. Breathing into the *tanden* is "right earthing," and opens the treasure of life.

> Sitting ... [into] the *Hara*-seat not only refers to the position and weight of the belly within the whole body but also suggests the whole mood of stable sitting. This stability implies at once an outward and an inward balance: it means that the inner center is situated in the right place in the physical body, as well as the right placing of the center of gravity within the body.... When the belly is sedate[7] the center is situated below (p. 57).

Breathing down into the vital center brings the breath deep into the diaphragm and brings energy into the regions below the diaphragm.

> Breathing is once more easy and free, and a pleasant feeling arises from below (p. 107).

7. In *New Webster's Dictionary and Thesaurus* (1992, p. 342), the word *sedate* translates into not excitable, composed, calm.

> What is necessary is a movement which leads downwards to the all-dissolving, all absorbing depth of the Source (p. 123).

How important can sitting meditation be for the pregnant women today, living with high levels of stress, a fast pace, and facing unknown circumstances?

> With [breathing into the] *Hara* the uprightness of the body is no longer the result of will and power but comes by itself. The whole body finds itself in flexible equilibrium. The difference in the tension of the neck is a special criterion of right posture. It is as if a secret power soared up lightly from below and culminated in the free carriage of the head. And so the letting go above gives concentration of strength below and the resulting easy freedom of the head has its counterpart in the sustaining weight of the trunk. Thus the practice of [breathing into the] *Hara* consists from the beginning in a constantly repeated letting go or dropping down movement. Then one notices how from the vital middle region strength rises straight upward through the back and produces the sensation of being uplifted (pp. 137–138).

Through the centuries, for pregnant women in both the Chinese and Japanese traditions, sitting meditation practice has offered remarkable birth enhancement. "The exercise of sitting is the most fundamental of all. Here the practice of stillness has its source. A thousand secrets are hidden in simply sitting still" (p. 142).

Sitting meditation is a superior means of prenatal care. It has important paranormal potential.

Feeding Elixir into the Womb Child[8]

MUCH ANCIENT WISDOM concerning the importance of deep breathing is contained in the *Zen* classic *The Embossed Tea Kettle* by the *Zen* Master Hakuin Zenji:

> As has been said by ancient wise men, the elixir is below the navel, the fluid is the fluid of the lungs, and one turns down the fluid of the lungs to the space below the navel, and so turns the lung fluid into the elixir (Zenji, 1963, p. 40).

The "fluid" in the lungs is the vital energy breathed into the body from the air,[9] "turned down" (breathed down) into the vital area below the navel. The language in Hakuin's writing is the language of medicine, of restoring and perfecting health. His indications were renowned for being effective. He continues:

> There are twelve kinds of breathings which help in curing all diseases. There is the rule about seeing a bean, as it were, below the navel. The purpose of doing so is to bring down the fire of the heart and concentrate it below the navel and right down to the soles of the feet. This not only cures diseases but helps greatly in Zen meditation (p. 41).

In this traditional wisdom of human function, the fluid energy breathed down into the vital lower abdominal area is seen to be stored there and is naturally retained (p. 67):

> There is what we call the "space below the abdomen" and this is the treasure room where the energy is stored and pre-

8. *Elixir* is defined by the *Webster's New World College Dictionary* as a remedy for all ailments.

9. Universal energy field (UEF), see Chapter III, Barbara Brennan.

served; here is the fortress town where the divine elixir is purified so that life may be preserved for long years.

When a pregnant woman practices breathing vital energy down to the child in her womb she brings the child elixir for greater function. The child will be blessed and the mother will probably be happy to maintain meditation practice, for her continued benefit, for the child, and for the benefit of those close to her. The child will probably be interested in meditation. This can be seen as the basis of a healthy society.

Secret Instructions

In the book *The Secret of the Golden Flower* by Richard Wilhelm, he speaks of the inner circulation of light and making breathing rhythmical. We might say that what he calls light is *chi*, vital energy. He says that the circulation of the light is in unison with the rhythms of breathing. The breath, the heart, and the light are interdependent. While in an upright sitting posture, an open channel is established that shifts the light downward, through the body, for circulation with the breath. This brings fine attention to the quality of breathing. There is more and more release in quieted consciousness.

True breathing, as Wilhelm refers to it, is then manifested in the quietness of the breath, when you become more conscious of the work of the heart. Then the movement form of the heart can be known. As the breathing is light, the heart is light. (Wilhelm seems to be combining the physical heart and the spiritual heart.) Breathing can help people focus into the heart for greater awareness.

The heart runs away easily, states Wilhelm, and it is necessary to center through the power of breathing. By refining the power of breathing, the heart becomes stable and quiet. Wilhelm addresses two mistakes of "quiet work": (1) laziness and (2) distraction. Sitting meditation posture will decrease distraction. Distraction often comes from letting the spirit wander aimlessly. Therefore, while sitting, it is helpful to keep the heart quiet with a concentrated attention and quiet breathing. The heart alone is conscious of the in- and outflowing of the breath. The true breath cannot be heard with the ears. Disciplined breath meditation removes laziness and can give a pregnant woman fuller use of her physical and energy bodies.

The Life Vase and the Womb

Among the various practices of Buddhist *Vajrayana* meditation, well received now in the West, lamas of the different lineages use the visualization of the Life Vase (Tibetan: *tse bum*), in the navel center. It has also been translated as the Vase of Immortality. The Life Vase is similar to or the same as both the *tan tien* and the *Hara*. There are no indications that these focal points for meditation are located inside of the physical womb in a woman. The physical and energy bodies are inseparable but different. They function at different frequencies of vibration. When a woman is pregnant her womb develops upward and moves toward the navel center, where the energetic Life Vase is located, in the energy body within the physical body.

When a pregnant woman breathes energy into her Life Vase, she feeds the development of the child's energy body in her womb. This practice is empowering. It helps women use inherent ability to experience new levels of function.

Pain-Body Release

A woman can bring a greater sense of her body into labor and delivery if she recognizes her pain-body. She can release centuries of accumulated fear that rises in childbirth. Eckhart Tolle writes about the woman and her pain-body in his book *The Power of Now:*

> The pain-body usually has a collective as well as a personal aspect. The personal aspect is the accumulated residue of emotional pain suffered in one's own past. The collective one is the pain accumulated in the collective human psyche over thousands of years through disease, torture, war, murder, cruelty, madness, and so on. Everyone's personal pain-body also partakes of this collective pain-body … every woman has her share in what could be described as the collective female pain-body. This consists of accumulated pain suffered by women partly through male subjugation of the female, through slavery, exploitation, rape, childbirth, child loss, and so on, over thousands of years.… Often, a woman is "taken over" by the pain-body … (Tolle, 1999, pp. 138–141).

This tends to be true during labor and delivery. The woman is apt to lose herself in the psychic pull of billions of women who have suffered cervical opening, and many thousands suffering at that moment, unless she has developed meditation awareness in preparation for labor. Then she may awaken to fully engage childbirth, alert to the pull of suffering, able to stay free by appreciating contraction pain, realizing greater function: "Do not let the pain-body use your mind and take over your thinking. Watch it. Feel its energy directly, inside your body. As you know, full attention means full acceptance" (p. 142).

Women have the inherent capacity to work with the pain-body and cervical opening. How they use this capacity is an educational challenge for society. Such education and the development it could inspire can reduce women's vulnerability in childbirth. It could reduce the need for drugs, anesthesia, and surgery in childbirth and improve the quality of health for all of society. When a woman in labor is aware of the collective pain-body and does not succumb to it, but sees it and frees it in the realization potential of labor, she can help free the species of its past and live its evolution. If she intends that, she can do that; and she can learn to intend that.

Practicing energy medicine for childbirth, women help safeguard the great potential of the human species and society.

V

The Calm Birth Methods

I know now that human beings are creatures of awareness, involved in an evolutionary journey of awareness, beings indeed unknown to themselves, filled to the brim with incredible resources that are never used . . .

—Carlos Castaneda, *Magical Passes*

Advanced Natural Childbirth

Practice of Opening: Healing the Nervous System for Prenatal Development

Womb Breathing: Expanded Childbirth Anatomy and Function

Giving and Receiving: The Potential of Healing in Childbirth

Instinctive Movement and Vocalization in Labor

Establishing an Effective Daily Practice

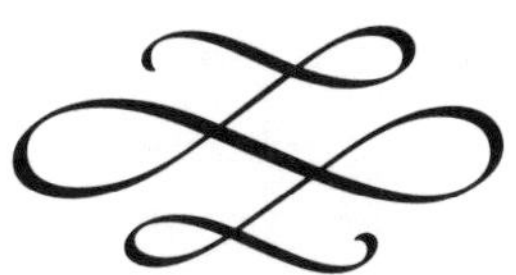

Advanced Natural Childbirth

IT IS TIME TO DELVE DEEP into the potential of childbirth methodology.

Advanced natural childbirth is an expression used to indicate childbirth with meditation methods designed specifically to advance childbirth methodology. Such methods should prove to have additional benefits beyond those described in Chapter II and may indicate deeper directions for childbirth research. Emerging childbirth methodology has the potential to give us high standards of maternal and infant health.

Calm Birth is an example of emerging childbirth methodology. Refined through ten years of development and application, the Calm Birth method includes three main techniques that work together. They are each derived from respected sources, with honored histories. In being applied to childbirth for the first time they offer new ranges of function to childbirth, enabling women to access their inherent potential for extraordinary experience in giving birth. The program also offers methods of instinctive and sacred movement. The Calm Birth methods are offered at a time when the large majority of women are willing to give up their potential for empowerment in birth because of fear of pain, fear of fear, and a culturally supported acceptance of giving birth numb from the waist down. That is a widely accepted abandonment of natural capability in which women don't have a chance to know what they can do naturally, often not even wanting to know their most distinctive capability. Calm Birth offers women the chance not only to command their remarkable normal ability to give birth, but to command even greater function and greater health whether they have a natural or a medicated birth. Calm Birth offers a chance to regain a sense of the sacred in giving birth. Intention is integral to the Calm Birth methods, intention to benefit all life by giving birth in a greater way.

Practice of Opening

Healing the Nervous System for Prenatal Development

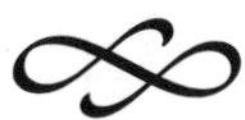

Introduction

The Calm Birth program is based on the clinical and research programs of the Harvard Medical School and the University of Massachusetts Medical Center (UMMC). In the UMMC program of medical meditation, designed to treat difficult medical cases in which pain management is an important concern, a combination of three methods has proven effective since 1979: reclining meditation, sitting meditation, and awareness-movement exercises. The Calm Birth program builds on the clinical success of the UMMC program by using four methods: reclining meditation, sitting meditation, a renowned healing practice, and instinctive and sacred movement.

Regarding the reclining meditation, UMMC uses the celebrated method of progressive relaxation (PR) developed by Edmund Jacobson, M.D., at the Harvard Medical School and the University of Chicago Medical School from the 1920s into the 1940s. The method enables neuromuscular release and a healing of the nervous system that has successfully treated various disease conditions. UMMC combines mindfulness-awareness meditation with PR, which makes the neuromuscular release more efficient. Calm Birth takes the neuromuscular release with mindfulness-awareness and modifies it for childbirth for the following purposes:

- to heal the nervous systems of woman and child in preparation for childbirth. The nervous system of the fetus may be healed of prenatal disturbances and organic conditions through sympathetic resonance with the woman's healed nervous system;
- to engage life force at the cellular level, to increase vitality in preparation for childbirth;
- to directly engage the womb child in energetic awareness in order to bring prenatal development to a new potential.

Description

The *Practice of Opening* is a reclining progressive relaxation meditation intended to bring the awareness of the woman and her partner into communion with the awareness of the unborn child, and to bring expanded capability and function into childbirth. Choose a quiet place dedicated to childbirth meditation. It can be the bedroom if necessary. Use blankets and pillows as needed to be comfortable. It's important to be at rest and alert with soft open eyes.

The audioguide helps the woman to be present in her body and feel fully capable. (Please see the audioguide narration that begins on page 47.) Beginning with sensing the cellular life force everywhere, her attention is directed to move progressively through her entire body, releasing neuromuscular stresses and reconditioning the nervous system. The muscle systems are progressively relaxed, taking pressure off the nervous system and the organs, allowing inner alignment and awakening in the woman and child. When a partner or other supporter joins in this practice, bonding with the child in the womb, the child's vital energy and awareness potentially increase.

Commentary

Progressive relaxation (PR) methods are various therapeutic techniques developed by Edmund Jacobson, M.D., in his more than three decades of medical practice. It's an early and valuable form of mind/body medicine. PR has provided impressive evidence of its effectiveness in successfully treating acute neuromuscular hypertension, chronic neuromuscular hypertension, states of fatigue and exhaustion, states of debility (convalescence from infectious and exhausting diseases of various types), organic and functional coronary disorders, chronic pulmonary tuberculosis, preoperative and postoperative conditions, toxic goiter, insomnia, various internal spasm conditions including cardio-spasm, and other conditions.

Dr. Jacobson saw that neuromuscular release therapy depended on patient self-initiative and nervous system reeducation. This was a breakthrough in noninvasive medicine and self-care, verging into new kinds of treatment. Jacobson developed extensive variations of PR in his medical practice.

In 1979, Jon Kabat-Zinn established the Mindfulness-Based Stress Reduction (MBSR) meditation program at the University of Massachusetts Medical Center (UMMC). The UMMC program uses a forty-five-minute reclining body scan to achieve progressive relaxation. Hundreds of American hospitals now use the UMMC reclining method with proven success. By combining mindfulness-awareness meditation with PR, this method encourages the mind to stay present, to stay valuably focused from moment to moment, maximizing the effectiveness of the practice. The body scan brings neuromuscular release and restoration. With respect to prenatal care, awareness-based PR offers a superior kind of relaxation meditation that may rectify existing conditions and enable women to realize new levels of life.

The Calm Birth program has expanded progressive relaxation for childbirth with an emphasis on developmental communion with the womb child and contact with life force at the cellular level. The *Practice of Opening* leads women through a process of neural reconditioning that prepares them for optimal function during delivery, for the realization of potential, and for the giving of life.

The *Practice of Opening* may produce extraordinary pre-birth experience (PBE) and near-birth experience (NBE), paranormal experience more accessible with this practice since awareness is less restricted by nervous stresses and is supported by hormonal enhancements as described in Chapter II.

Key Points

- The *Practice of Opening* childbirth method offers rest, restoration, and release for increased natural capability during labor and delivery.
- Relaxing neuromuscular tensions and rectifying conditions caused by stress deepen physical confidence and awareness.
- In doing the *Practice of Opening* a woman may solve longstanding health challenges while she maintains superior prenatal care.
- This method can bring the pregnant woman and her partner to healing and a healthful union with the child, an awareness cohesion that should enhance the child's intelligence.
- *Body Light:* The atoms of the human body contain high-speed electrons that leave brilliant traces of light. Our dynamic atoms are locked magnetically in powerful molecules, all bright with light. The experience of light may be one of our earliest experiences. In the *Practice of Opening* we directly engage the body of light in our body of cells as a prenatal resource.
- The *Practice of Opening* is intended to give women a method of empowerment and personal development, to help them find the realization potential of childbirth so much needed today, in the circumstance where prevalent childbirth education is not interested in this inherent potential.
- Childbirth has often been a time of extraordinary experiences for women, including paranormal spiritual experiences. The *Practice of Opening* encourages such events.

Practice of Opening

(the practice)

THE FOLLOWING IS A TRANSCRIPT of the audioguide transmission of this method. You can read this transcription and understand its intention. You can also obtain the audioguide CD and experience the method through audioguidance. If you are pregnant, the womb child will be responsive to the audioguidance.

Introduction

The *Practice of Opening* is a reclining meditation.
It offers a way to progressively relax and open your body,
releasing stress on your nerves,
healing your nervous system.
The womb child is responsive to meditation
in both mother and father.
This practice is a chance to come into greater awareness,
to enliven you and your child.
You're a woman holding new life dynamically alive in your womb,
or you're a man who wants to benefit your partner and child
by imagining the womb in yourself.
With this practice you learn to rest and release,
gaining vital force and new function.

Please find a comfortable place to rest
and lie down mindfully, using pillows as needed.
It's important to be comfortable and warm.
This practice is done with soft open eyes
so that you don't fall asleep.
The effects are immediate, and they build over time.
You'll benefit the most with daily practice.
Whenever you need to rest, this is an ideal way
to calm and open your body
and enter the life force in your cells.

The Practice

Please take a deep breath, deep into life, and exhale slowly.
Feel life energy in all of your body at once.
Again breathe deep into life, and exhale slowly.
Let yourself experience total body sensation.
Feel the billions of cells and energy pathways.

Please imagine the dynamics of your central nervous system,
taking care of countless functions at once.
Messages travel quickly to and from your developing child.
Rest, and understand that as you become
aware of living light in you,
you directly benefit the child in your womb.
From head to toes feel your body's flow.
Experience the enlivening of your child.
Feel that the new life in you is unlimited.
Feel the living presence of your child.

As your awareness expands
take time to relax, slowly and deeply, resting in union.
Soon you'll be guided to focus part by part into your body,
to release all that needs to be released.
As you breathe, open and sense all the life moving
in you and your child.
Every time you return to this awareness
you feel great internal life support.
Feel the forces creating life in you, sustaining life in you.
Recognize the miracle of life you are,
and the miracle of life being created in you,
the child in your womb.

Now notice the toes of both your feet.
Experience the life in your toes.
Feel their energy channels.
Feel the energy channels in your feet.
Throughout your feet notice how the bones give stability and form.
Sense how your feet serve you in many ways.
If there's any discomfort, notice where.
Breathe into it and release as much as you can.
Feel the total current of life in your feet.

Move your attention up into the calves of both your legs.
Notice the muscle system and nerves.
Sense how the muscles, nerves, and blood flow all work together.
Throughout your feet and lower legs,
feel and release more muscles and nerves.
Feel an increase of vitality in your lower legs and feet.
Now become aware of your knees.
Notice life force flowing through them.
This is a good way to meditate, reclaiming your body,
knowing your body as if for the first time, a body alive with child.
From your knees, come up into your thighs.
Feel how your living thighs support and carry your body.
Notice and release any tension in your buttocks.
Recognize their power to support you in childbirth.
Breathe into those muscles and feel body fluids circulate.
All throughout your feet, legs, and hips,
feel the smaller and larger bones,
muscles, . . . blood vessels, . . . and nerves.
Feel it all together.
Release any holding.
Feel the energy gain and sense the life flow.
As you feel your body and your child more and more
you both become more alive.
It is time to bond directly.
Place your hands lightly on your belly.
Be sensitive to the life of your child.
Feel the life force in you both.
Come into new life in your self and your child.
Release any block to the full flow of life.
Enter greater awareness.
Sense the power and wisdom of your child.
If you feel tension, breathe into it, and give it space.
Breathe into and out of any areas of discomfort or pain.

Practice of Opening

Please relax more and more.
Feel both of your arms full of life.
Feel the life force moving through your arms and hands.
Rest your wrists and relax your hands.
Feel their healing ability.
Imagine their potential to care for your child.
Relaxing your arms down through your fingers,
breathe care into the child,
trusting the process of life.
Feel your womb and cervix holding your child.
At the right time, your womb will start to flex
and your cervix will begin to respond,
slowly opening, progressively releasing new life.
The baby's head will then move down through the birth canal.
The pelvis will work with the womb
when you breathe the baby down to be born.
Feel the strength and flexibility of your womb,
yielding to growth and change.
These are the strongest muscles in your body,
fully capable of birthing your baby.
Relax any abdominal tension caused by anxiety.
Practice relaxing the outer and inner muscles that cradle your child.
Surrender into the full support of life.
Trust your ability to change.
Prepare to give birth to your child.

Now, turning your focus to your baby, envision your child's head,
facial features,... torso,... arms and legs,... muscles,... organs.
See your child's heart pulsing blood all through its body,
feeding its cells with radiant life.
It's time to feel the nurturing flow of your organs
and the energetic organs of your child.

Feel the flow of life in your flesh,
and be sensitive to life energy in the child.
Trust the living wisdom in you both.
Now please turn your attention to the umbilical cord and placenta,
vibrant with thousands of body processes.
Imagine the energy flowing in the lifelines of the cord,
back and forth between your child's body
and your nurturing placenta.
All around all this is the cradling womb.
Once again feel your whole body
deeper and more completely than ever.
Breathe awareness into your belly.
Breathe easily and deep,
bringing in oxygen and energy.
As you breathe out, gently contract your belly inward,
caressing your child.
Recognize any abdominal tension from anxiety restricting your breath.
Let the muscles there release. Trust the flow of life.
Completely open yourself to your body.
Completely open yourself to your baby.
Completely open yourself to life.
Breathe easily and deeply.

Please bring your attention into your upper body.
Relax the muscles through your ribcage and chest.
Notice any fear.
Please recognize and release any apprehension.
Trust your ability and strength.
Open your shoulders and chest.
Breathe in deeply, and relax as you breathe out.
Feel your breasts coming alive with milk.
Know that your breasts are vital for your child.

As you continue breathing with awareness,
enter the dynamic majesty of your heart.
Recognize all that the heart does to maintain life.
Intuit your heart's four-fold pulsing rhythm.
It beats for every cell in you and your child.
Your heart sustains your lives.
Open into pulsing union.
Rest in pulsing union.

Bring your focus to your back.
Let your spine extend.
Feel bones and connective tissue adjust.
The life force in your spine
carries you and your child.
Please bring your awareness up your spine,
through your shoulders into your neck.
Open and let sensation flow.
The stress of demands of the day
tends to be held in the neck and spine.
Please unlock and release these demands.
Let yourself be free right now.
Please relax the front of your neck and open your throat.
Feel your breath flowing in,... and flowing out.

Now, become aware of your face.
Breathe into your jaw letting it loosen.
Notice the different sets of muscles around your mouth,
forming expressions both conscious and unconscious.
Find all these muscles and relax them,
releasing all expression.
Let your mouth open a little
and release any holding in your lower face and neck.
Relax your tongue and silently flow.
Coming to your eyes and the muscles that surround them,

sense all the expression they have,
all the expression of your life.
Relax all that completely. Let it go.
Prepare to feel empowered giving birth.
Let your face be free right now.
Resting with soft open eyes,
your energized body prepares.
This is a master path.

To conclude this practice,
know that you've empowered yourself and your child.
Live in this awareness as you move.

Womb Breathing

Expanded Childbirth Anatomy and Function

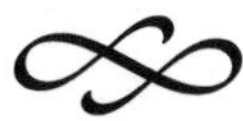

Introduction

Womb Breathing is energy breathing for childbirth. Energy breathing has been known and used for centuries, but it's never been offered to women as an evolutionary childbirth method. During the history of our planet, in various cultures, traditions of meditation science developed in which breathing energy into the navel center in the energy body was a key feature. That was known to have great value for realization and evolution. The directive to breathe energy into the navel center was given regardless of sexual gender. Practitioners were predominantly men. Women were generally not expected to be interested in doing such practice, and were probably not encouraged to do so. But in some instances, such as in the *Nyingma* lineage of Tibetan Buddhism, women and men were equally encouraged to do such practice.

Today, with the evolutionary quality of our species impacted by the widespread use of drugs and anesthesia in childbirth, the use of meditation practice based on breathing energy into the navel center for prenatal care may be the most valuable application of the practice ever. Women who practice *Womb Breathing* are aware that their practice raises the quality of two lives, inseparably; and through the intention that their practice may benefit as many people as possible, the practice is being used with deeper implication and potential than ever. The intention to benefit other people with meditation practice, and to benefit as many people as possible, is also a feature of *Giving and Receiving*.

Description

Womb Breathing is a classic sitting meditation practice based on a profound energy breathing technique proven effective for centuries. The practice works through respect for innate capabilities of the human multidimensional body and its extraordinary breathing potential. The practice of *Womb Breathing* changes the nature and quality of breathing and the nature and quality of psychophysical function, with important benefit for the child.

Psychologically, the practice is based on recognizing the difference between mind and awareness. This is mindfulness-awareness meditation in which women learn to recognize mind, to see how laden with anxiety and fear it is, and to see that much of the fear and anxiety is not their own. Women who practice this method become progressively more able to recognize and release fear. *Womb Breathing* is a greater kind of breathing as a basis of greater physiological and psychological function.

Daily prenatal practice of this sitting meditation enables a deeper kind of breathing that takes place effortlessly beyond the practice period, throughout the course of the day and night, because the body likes to function at the more optimal levels it was designed for. With the direct development of fearlessness facilitated by this practice, women are offered a complete vision of body/mind health in childbirth. This is the most essential of the three Calm Birth prenatal methods because it is a transformative breathing method that, with practice, may come spontaneously at any time, and may be of great value to women throughout the labor process. This sitting practice is based on visualization.

Visualization

> Imagery practice can give rise to meta-normal powers and consciousness by the recruitment of many somatic processes. Through such recruitment, countless cells are somehow enlisted by mental images so that as an integral whole they support extraordinary functioning (Leonard and Murphy, 1995, p. 115).

Visualization is a transformative modality. Visualization of our body systems, such as our energy body systems, can help people see the way to extraordinary functioning.

If we visualize a pregnant woman's body as a multidimensional breathing body, sitting to meditate, we can see her inseparable physical and energy bodies. In her fully envisioned breathing facilities we can see her lungs and a luminous Life Vase, very near her womb, but in a different dimension. The Life Vase is an important feature of the energy body in both women and men. It's made for a profound kind of breathing, to strengthen life force.

When a pregnant woman is practicing *Womb Breathing,* it may look like she's breathing into her womb, but actually she's breathing into her Life Vase to benefit the womb child. She's using her full breathing capability, breathing with her physical body and her energy body at once. With *Womb Breathing* the woman uses her lungs fully, with abdominal breathing for full oxygenation, and she's using her energy body by breathing energy into her Life Vase. The energy breathed feeds up into her central psychic channel, bringing greater function to the woman and the child in her womb.

As a woman spends more time engaged in the *Womb Breathing* practice, she can visualize and see her energy body more completely. It consists of countless energy channels, ranging in size from the large central psychic channel, with its radiant series of power centers, to small fine conduits. She can see that her central channel rises from the bottom of the Life Vase, which is made for breathing vital energies from the air into the central channel, to balance the energy centers and bring higher systems to life. This increased inner activity benefits the child in the womb through the child's neurohormones and sympathetic resonance, an energetic response to the woman's energy uptake.

The whole system of channels is dynamic, and has been seen and used by energy science and meditation science in different cultures for more than two thousand years. There are subtle channels that quickly pulse into and out of existence, depending on the energy states of the individual. The central energy channel with its brilliant power centers has energetic correspondence to the central nervous system as the Life Vase corresponds to the womb.

The energy body Life Vase is located behind the physical navel, between four finger widths above the navel to four finger widths below. The central channel rises from the bottom of the Vase up to the crown *chakra* located in the top of the head. The conscious breathing of both bodies into dynamic cohesion is based on practical knowledge refined over many centuries, knowledge of breathing energy from the air into the Life Vase in the navel center, "the transformation center." This knowledge can help transform natural childbirth.

Womb Breathing is *Vase Breathing* practiced by a pregnant woman. She knows that the Life Vase and the womb are close. She knows that the deep breathing practice benefits the womb child energetically, biologically, and psychologically.

To visualize what is breathed, the woman senses that the air she lives in is in a universal energy field (UEF). The UEF is presently an important subject of scientific inquiry, but it has been recognized and utilized for more than two thousand years by venerable meditation science traditions. It's been called universal *chi* and universal *prana*.[10] Scientists today call it bio-plasma, the basis of living matter (see Chapter III). The UEF is known to be omnipresent vital energy, and we're made to breathe it down into the Life Vase. It has a fundamental affinity for the life in our bodies. Inside the energy body, flowing in its channels, is the same fundamental vital energy.

The external *chi* can be seen by some people but is mostly sensed intuitively. As Castaneda suggests (see Chapter IV), women may sense it more quickly than men. Most people live their lives breathing it in and breathing it out without sensing or using it.

---

10. "The word *prana* is derived from the Sanskrit word meaning 'absolute energy.' *Prana* is the principal element, the vital force that distinguishes living entities from inanimate objects.... According to the ancient masters, *prana* is the mystical force that is found in all living physical entities but which is nonphysical. It is in air without being air. It ... can be experienced, or felt ..." (Khalsa and Stauth, 2001, p. 55).

It's important to recognize this energy and intentionally breathe it. To begin, it's important to sense it. It's possible to feel breathing it down into the Life Vase directly by breathing it and intending it down into the Life Vase. From the Life Vase it absorbs up into the central channel for increased mind/body function.

First the woman senses the energy and the Life Vase. She may or may not ever see them. The Life Vase is inside her and the energy is in the air she breathes. The woman visualizes and senses that in the region of the womb in another dimension is a Life Vase, a luminous breathing Vase for strengthening life force. She breathes into her Life Vase for the sake of the child in her womb. This is new childbirth anatomy. This is a method with a vision of what the woman's body was made to do, a vision of the potential of natural childbirth.

According to meditation science the pineal gland, associated with the crown *chakra,* may be discerned in the human embryo as early as the moment of conception, the time that the basis of the navel *chakra* is also formed. According to the direct experience of Tibetan meditation masters who passed through death into rebirth with undisturbed awareness, in the moment of conception the sperm ("father seed essence") does not merge completely with the egg ("mother seed essence"). Both the egg and sperm retain a brilliant fragment of their original identity and hold a dynamic polar field of connection with each other, forming the basis of the energy body. The father seed essence will become the crown *chakra* and the mother seed essence will become the navel *chakra,* radiantly white and red, respectively (Sogyal, 1994, p. 254). Thus knowledge that is considered sacred states that the energy body forms simultaneously with the physical body from conception.

Seeing the energy body as integral to the physical body, the woman breathes with dynamic vision, breathes with two bodies, for her own sake, for the child, for her family, and for the greater good.

Posture

To experience the full benefit of *Womb Breathing,* it's important to sit so that the body is upright, comfortable, and balanced, on a cushion or in a chair. Sit with great respect for all the dimensions of life in the body. Some people sit cross-legged, using a cushion to lift the pelvis and sacrum a little, so the body weight is distributed evenly. The spine should be as upright as possible, balanced, and at ease; it may tend to lift a little, effortlessly. When sitting in a chair, both feet are placed flat on the floor directly in front of the body. Hands are placed on the knees, or held softly together in the lap.

Sitting upright and balanced is the best posture for *Womb Breathing*. The woman can shift into spontaneous *Womb Breathing* in any posture, but sitting is the best posture for sustained, effective practice. It encourages coming to still-point to shift to awareness of the energy body. Sitting to come into greater function enables people to calm down their minds, to bring the center of gravity of intensive functioning down to the vital center, to shift attention from mind to inherent open awareness. Awareness is still and open and able to see fear and other emotions without attaching to them. Sitting meditation helps calm the body and mind for greater psychophysical function.

Breathing

All our life we've breathed energy in and out, absorbing it inadequately. The absorption is potentially under our control. Revered ancient yogic texts call the external energy in the breath *prana* (*pra* = first unit; *na* = energy). Internal *prana* "is the most subtle unit of [life] energy and it is organized into . . . [an] energy field, which underlies the physical structure and functioning of the body and is potentially under the control of the mind" (Rama, 1979, p. xii).

"The physical body is a crystallization around the energy body that underlies it" (p. 130). This energy body "has an extremely complex 'anatomy,' comprised of certain pathways called nadis [channels] through which the pranic energy [breath] flows" (pp. 10–11). "The flow of breath [prana] is constantly shaping the pattern of energy flow that underlies and sustains the physical body" (p. 12). "Of the five major pranas, one of them is the energy that governs the breath" (p. 93).

In *Womb Breathing, prana* energy in the air is sensed, and tension in the body is relaxed as much as possible. *Prana* in the body governs the breathing of *prana* into the body. The external *prana,* vital life energy of the universe, has a fundamental affinity for the body, but if that isn't recognized the energy is poorly absorbed. In *Womb Breathing* that energy is recognized, breathed in, and intended directly into the Life Vase, for all the energy systems. It absorbs into the womb child energetically, strengthening the child's life.

This fine, deep, slow breathing is oxygen rich as well as energy rich. It's fine breathing because it senses and extracts fine substance from the air. It's deep breathing because it uses full breathing capability and brings the breath in deep, into the energy body. It's slow breathing because the increased intake requires fewer breaths per minute, expending less energy, increasing and extending life.

Whatever posture the woman is in, it is important for her to breathe completely, using her chest and belly and Vase, knowing she's developing her ability to be fully capable in labor and delivery, breathing in a greater way. This kind of breathing can inspire women to be more present and aware and to free themselves of obstructive emotions carried by the mind.

Commentary

Womb Breathing is closely based on the *Vajrayana* Buddhist (Tibetan) meditation method called *Vase Breathing* (*Bum Chung,* Tib.). *Prana* (*lung,* Tib.; *chi,* Ch.), meaning air, wind, or vital energy, is breathed into the Life Vase in the navel center. There are practices in the yogic traditions of India and the Taoist tradition of China of breathing *prana* or *chi* down into the navel center. Because of the presence of Tibetan meditation masters in Europe and America for the past thirty years, the meditation practice of *Bum Chung, Vase Breathing,* has been available for use in childbirth in the West from an authoritative living tradition widely available.

The phrase "energy body" was popularized by Carolyn Myss, Ph.D., in her best-selling book *Anatomy of the Spirit* (1996). Myss, a "medical intuitive," sees the energy body as having the salient features of a central energy channel with a vertical series of seven "*chakras*," energy power wheels. She "saw" that this vision of the energy body was similar in each of the major religions. Her work has influenced the medical science trend to consider extended anatomy.

In the profound *Vajrayana* Buddhist meditation tradition, which it seems Myss was not informed of, much detail is given on the form and function of the energy body. Importantly, a breathing Vase is known to be located in the naval center, from which the integral central psychic channel rises. Extensive detail of the channel systems and the function of *Vase Breathing* is transmitted in *Vajrayana* Buddhist meditation. It is this instruction that the *Womb Breathing* meditation practice is based on.

If it's true, as Don Juan Matus said, that in the Toltec knowledge women have an advantage in seeing energy, then a woman's inherent ability to see energy may be her special skill for *Womb Breathing* meditation. Women may have a natural superiority in meditation when the practice is based on sensing and breathing vital energy from the air. If a woman at first doesn't see the *prana,* the living substance in the air, she can trust that it's there and she can breathe it. We are made to breathe energy.

In advanced physical science, open space itself is seen to be full of energy, an energy bank from which the universe evolves. It may be in several states at one time. This fundamental energy pervading all space is the omnipresent medium that perennial wisdom says is breathable.

Why is the omnipresent energy medium breathable? If that external energy is also the fundamental life energy in the human body, we're made to breathe the external UEF because there's a natural affinity between the internal and external UEF. We're made to breathe vital energy in the air to strengthen vital force in the energy body.

A woman can learn to practice *Womb Breathing* while she sleeps, to benefit the womb child while she sleeps. This instruction is given in the Calm Birth teacher certification program.

Partners in the birth, and midwives, nurses, doctors, and doulas, can practice breathing energy into their Life Vase to be supportive, imagining that child in their body. Both the pregnant woman and her womb child can sensitively receive the beneficial energy of such intention. This kind of breathing inspires greater awareness and psychological freedom. When a partner is supportively doing the practice, this unified prenatal team can take childbirth to a new potential.

Energy breathing quiets the body and can bring relative calm into labor and delivery. The practice can help women be open, aware, and relatively calm in contractions and in the intervals between contractions. *Womb Breathing* women may experience grace in the face of contraction pain. They may demonstrate childbirth without fear and without suffering. Some of the women go through labor and never forget the child or the Life Vase. *Womb Breathing* works with *Giving and Receiving* during contractions to give a two-fold basis of breathing into contractions (see below).

The woman who develops meditation skills for childbirth may be learning meditation for the rest of her life. Childbirth can open the path of meditation. After childbirth *Womb Breathing* becomes *Vase Breathing,* for postnatal care and healing, and for an ongoing practice of transformative body and breathing.

Sacred Movements

In the Calm Birth teacher training program people learn a series of ennobling movements that formally establish sacred breathing in sacred body. Even though people can spontaneously engage *Womb Breathing* at any time, sitting, moving, or reclining, when sitting to begin the *Womb Breathing* practice it is best to begin with the series of sacred movements *(mudras),* to come directly into full potential, to sit into your body as if you're sitting into life itself. The *Womb Breathing mudras* are a graceful series of movements loaded with realization that there is inherent aware freedom from emotion and thought, and you can dispel, break the spell, in which emotion and thought often hold you. With a series of empowering movements people practice dispelling patterns of thought and emotion that limit human function. Acting from an internal ground of psychological freedom in which people can recognize and release emotions and thoughts that reduce human ability, women who practice these movements will increase their ability to see and dissolve fears that may arise during the process of labor. They know their inner freedom and source of psychological strength.

Controlled Release

In the traditional teaching of *Vase Breathing (Bum Chung)* in *Vajrayana* Buddhism, people are asked to practice a gentle retaining of the energy breathed down into the Vase. Traditionally people practice breathing energy down into the Vase and then holding it briefly, for two or three seconds. They release the exhale before the retention feels uncomfortable. We have changed that a little with respect to pregnant women. We ask people to practice a controlled release, breathing energy effortlessly down into the Vase, at ease in the normal cycle of breath, and then exhaling a little more slowly than that, as slow as feels comfortable. Exhaling the Vase breath more slowly than it is inhaled is practicing a gentle retaining of the vital energy. If there is the slightest discomfort or strain the exhale can be immediately released. Practicing *Vase Breathing* for pregnancy *(Womb Breathing),* with controlled release the woman has the instant ability to release the energy breath if the sensation of discomfort arises. She can retain the energy breath as much as she wants to by spontaneously regulating how slow or fast she wants to exhale. It is effortless to exhale a little more slowly than one inhales without disturbing the natural cycle of the breath. When the body is doing *Vase Breathing* on its own, naturally, it may gently retain the energy breath by exhaling more slowly than it inhales, giving the energy breathed into the Vase more time to absorb up into the central energy channel.

Benefits of Womb Breathing

1. Energy Increase

Womb Breathing sitting meditation saves energy, restores energy, and absorbs vital energy, giving birthing women greater function and clarity for fetal development, labor, and delivery.

Sitting meditation prevents wasteful expenditure of energy in the ceaseless activity of life, giving women a method to stop the external action and calm down.

In sitting meditation, energy reserves that may be run-down from high activity levels begin to restore. Research has proven that meditation is significantly better than sleep in restoring and increasing energy (Pelletier, 1977).

With *Womb Breathing,* women learn to shift frequently from mind to open awareness, saving vital energy that would be lost in the activity of mind. Mind burns up psychic energy. The willful feeding of energy to the mind is a primary cause of fatigue and burnout. *Womb Breathing* sitting meditation helps a woman free herself from the anxious action of the mind by repeatedly returning to open awareness, saving energy needed for greater function. Using a sitting meditation method to reduce the force of mind, women can come to intuitive wisdom and maximize capability for childbirth.

The shallow breathing prevalent in active people is inefficient, resulting in oxygen limitation and fatigue. It takes up to seven times more energy to breathe badly, overusing intercostal (between the ribs) muscles. *Womb Breathing* is effortless deep breathing, bringing in oxygen-plus with no energy cost.

With this more complete use of the human ability to breathe, a pregnant woman has the potential to give herself and her child the energy needed for vital health and full capability. The universe is an endless source of energy, immediately available. For those who want to intentionally breathe life energy, for those who want to breathe life force into the fetus within, universal vital energy has always been present for us to use.

2. Breathing into Contractions

Often women stop breathing and hold their breath during contractions, or are directed to do shallow, high-chest "pant-blow" breathing, which is like hyperventilation. That technique is admittedly useful at one critical juncture during labor, when it is desirable to stop an overwhelming impulse to push at the point of crowning, in order to allow the perineal tissues to stretch to prevent tearing. Other than in this case, both holding the breath and hyperventilation may cause fear by correspondence since anxiety and fear most often cause people to hold their breath or to limit it to shallow rapid breathing. This inhibits both physiological and psychological function.

Breathing fully into contractions, something women are capable of but are rarely encouraged to do, tends to reduce or eliminate the occurrence of fear, and gives them a positive, willed action to perform while the body continues the process of labor. Fear of pain intensifies the sensations and causes the body to work against itself through neuromuscular tension, thereby prolonging labor and often being the cause of medical intervention. Breathing into contractions reduces the incidence of fear and medical intervention so that women can access their full range of capability in labor.

After practicing the shift from mind to awareness with *Womb Breathing* throughout pregnancy, women in labor tend to spontaneously breathe into contractions. As a woman recognizes fear and frees herself to breathe, freeing her body to do its work, contraction pain is transformed as she breathes into it.

Following is a description by Gay Hendricks of a birth he attended that demonstrated the innate capacity of a woman to breathe into contractions:

> ... The laboring woman used her breath to breathe into the contractions, participating with the sensations rather than fighting them. By doing so she was able to transform the pain. Later she said it was never painful while she was using her breath. Sometimes a contraction would start as pain, but as she remembered to breathe into it, a shift would occur: Pain would become sensation (Hendricks, 1995, p. 19).

Clearly it's possible to breathe into contractions and stay calm in the process. A daily practice of meditation supports this response. Awareness enables women to recognize and dispel anxiety and fear. Then when labor begins, whatever pain is experienced can be recognized as the body performing its most marvelous function: birthing a new human being. Women who meditate are able to open instinctively to the sensations of their body in labor, to avoid suffering, and to come into full function in the creation of life. "We cannot labor with our intellect. We women need to reclaim this animal part of us and embrace ancient and necessary wisdom.... Once settled in, women in labor, then, must *allow* the pain" (Northrup, 1988, pp. 483 and 485). The instinctive shift from mind to awareness in labor—a shift developed in meditation practice—frees women of the restrictions of the intellect, and returns them to profound inner resources. Breathing into the contractions, staying with the sensations, women tend to experience sacred illumination in giving birth.

3. Recognition and Release of Fear in Contractions

The key to calm in contractions is adequate preparation in self-calming practices, such as *Womb Breathing*, on a daily basis, until the woman is prepared to see and let go of fear as it arises.

The more one practices psychological meditation such as *Womb Breathing*, the more one exposes mind to awareness. The mind is slowly revealed. There are many aspects to the mind, one's own ordinary thinking, memories, and projections, but the aspects of the mind that can be used for human development are anxiety and fear. Particularly with respect to childbirth, when anxiety and fear can result in risky medical interventions that may impair fetal and/or maternal health, it is vital for women to know that they have methods available through which they can expose their anxieties and fear in preparation for childbirth, and in doing so experience joy and release.

Centuries of experience with meditation practices such as *Womb Breathing* have shown that we have the innate capacity to recognize anxiety and fear in its various forms, and to work with them. The more we practice meditation the more we know the varieties of anxiety and fear. Facing fear is transformative.

> The willingness to face fear is itself fearlessness. Fearlessness is not merely the numb absence of fear. It is the strength and dignity that are nourished each time we face fear directly ... the strength that comes from directly stepping into fear.... Each time you go directly through the gateway of fear, you touch a more profound level of fearlessness and genuine confidence (Hayward and Hayward, 2001, p. 67).

Facing fear changes its quality. That doesn't necessarily dispel it. But daily practice of mindfulness-awareness breathing meditation, such as *Womb Breathing*, makes it inevitable that women anticipate and see their fears. They see that many of the fears within them are not their own, but come from the collective unconscious mind, as revealed by Jung (see Tolle, Chapter IV). Fears that are more personally their own are recognized as such and are energetically changed in that moment. Sometimes that's enough to dispel them.

The more we're aware of our mind, aware of our thoughts, the more we know we are not our thoughts. The more we're aware of our anxieties, the more we know we are not our anxieties. The more we're aware of our fears, the more we know we are not our fears. The woman who practices meditation for prenatal care is able to see and release fears that arise in labor, to free herself and feel the species begin to heal.

Learning the Practice

Learning to sense and breathe energy in the air and intend it down into the Life Vase can be compared to learning to ride a bicycle when you were a child. At first it may have seemed difficult—balancing on the bike, using the pedals, and moving ahead all at once—but seeing that all the other children readily learned how to do it was encouraging. Countless thousands of people have done energy breathing, for centuries, and now more and more people are doing it around you as the interest in meditation grows. Sensing that you were made to do it, when you first breathe energy and intend it down into the Vase and feel it go into the Vase, you know it's natural and you're beginning to get the knack.

Calm Labor

Womb Breathing the Night of the Birth

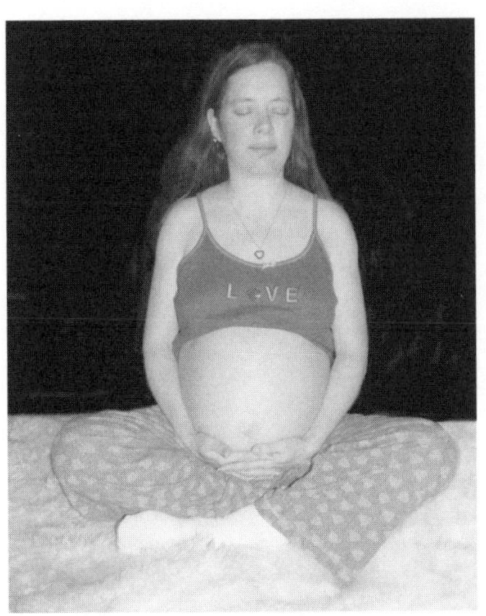

Debbie at 5 cm dilation

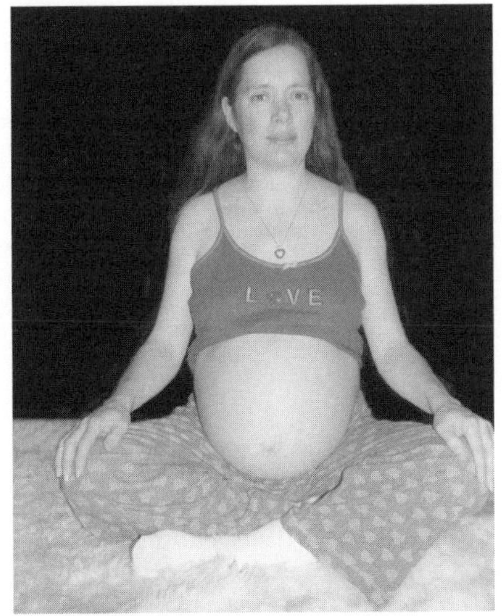

Debbie at 6 cm dilation

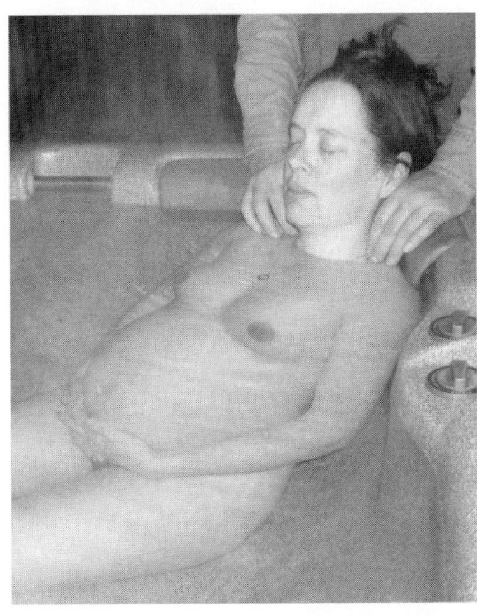

Debbie in tub, 9 cm dilation
(an hour before the birth)

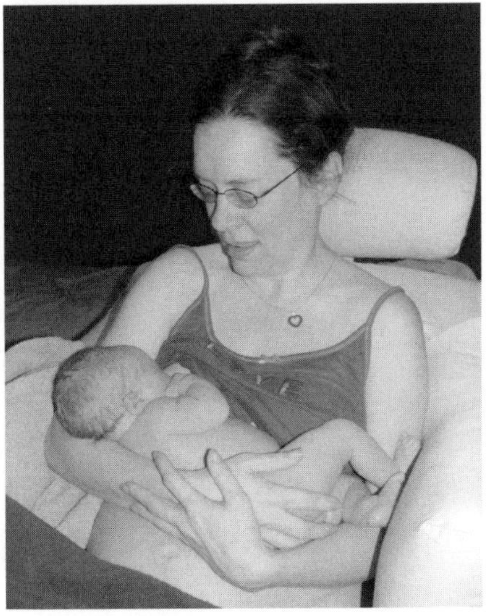

Happy birthday!

Womb Breathing

(the practice)

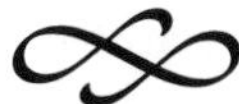

THE FOLLOWING IS A TRANSCRIPT of the audioguide transmission of this method. You can read this transcription and understand its intention. You can also obtain the audioguide CD and experience the method through audioguidance. If you are pregnant, the womb child will be responsive to the audioguidance.

Womb Breathing is energy breathing for childbirth.
It gives you deep body and greater function.
Womb Breathing helps you free yourself from fear.
This method is from meditation science.
While sitting, you learn to breathe energy into your energy body.
You do it to free yourself and feed
vital energy to the child in your womb.
You're made to breathe vital energy from the air.
You're made to feed vital energy to the child in your womb.

By sitting to calm and breathe in a deeper way
you can help your self and your child.
So please sit, as upright as possible, comfortable and at ease.
See that there's a luminous breathing Vase
in the navel center in your energy body.
It's a very soft Vase,
a radiant Vase.
It's called the Vase of Life.
It's known and respected in different traditions.
Sense that you're made to breathe vital energy into the Vase.
Sense that all your life you've been breathing energy in the air,
breathing it in and out without using it.
In order to breathe it in and down into the Vase
you need to intend the energy in and down.
When you do you'll feel it go into the Vase.
Practice breathing energy from the air down into the Vase.

As you continue to breathe energy into the Vase of Life
it absorbs up into your energy body channels.
Your child resonates with this energy,
becoming more alive.

Please do this sitting practice for at least twenty minutes in the morning.

Womb Breathing

Play the CD for audioguidance,
and then practice for a few minutes a few times a day.
Your body likes to do the practice.
You do *Womb Breathing* naturally.
The more you do it the more it happens instinctively.
The more you practice, the more this breathing
will emerge spontaneously during labor.
Please do it now.
Breathe energy from the air into your Vase of Life.

Sit with effortless upright balance on the floor with cushions,
or sit in a chair if that's easier for you.
Sit upright into your body as if you're sitting into life itself.
Sit and breathe life into your Vase for your child.

Shift your body a little if you need to.
Find your balance and breathe easily into your energy body.
Breathe with your belly and the Life Vase in your navel.
Sense the energy of the universal field all around you, supporting you.
Breathe into it gently and deeply.
Realize that you're made to use that energy to breathe in a greater way.
Engage the total sensation of your body,
your physical body and your energy body.
Feel yourself breathe completely.
Appreciate the many dimensions of life in you and your unborn child.
Breathe in a way that will give you and your child greater life.
Gain a sense of sacred body as you breathe in a deeper way.
With this breathing a child can be born free of fear.
Learn to breath-feed your energy body.
Allow yourself to absorb vital energy from the air.
Learn to breath-feed your child.

Breathe vital essence from the air into your energy body and your child.

You're a billion-fold system of energy pathways.
You have a central energy channel with brilliant centers, alive with light.
You have an energy breathing Vase in your navel center.
You have a body for a greater kind of birth.
You can give your child advantage, and life gain.
So please, sit and breathe in this way.
Breathe with open awareness.
Learn to sense the life-giving energy field all around you.
Breathe energy of the universal life force.
Learn to support yourself in a greater way with what's available.
Know your energy body.
Breathe vital energy.
Breathe into the Vase.
Breathe life into your Vase for your child.

As you remain comfortably upright, breathing slow and deep,
notice how your mind distracts you.
You may find you're lost in thought,
no longer aware of breathing vital energy.
You lose that intention.
You may be thinking about something that happened,
or thinking about something that's going to happen.
You may be anxious about something and you're not present.
Then something wakes you up.
Your awareness wakes you up to breathe with intention.
Breathe universal energy, vital life-giving energy.
Slow down and go deep.
See how your mind may take you away,
and then your awareness wakes you up and brings you back.
Continue breathing vital energy.

Don't identify with thoughts that come up.
Don't identify with emotions.
Stay with energy breathing in bodily calm and open awareness.
Breathe energy easily.
Breathe into the Vase.
Breathe life into the Vase.
Feel the energy you breathe absorb into your body.
Feel the energy absorb into your child.
Feel how you both gain life.

During the practice, fears may arise in different ways,
causing anxious thoughts distracting you from being present.
It's important to recognize anxiety and fear.
Catch your fears and they tend to dissolve.
Return to awareness of energy breathing.
It's a matter of life.
Come to life.
Breathe life.

See that you can do this with ease.
Come into new function, with living awareness.
When you breathe this way, it helps you free yourself from thought.
It helps you free yourself from fear.
Breathe into your energy body.
Feel the energy gain.
Practice day and night.
Practice in your sleep.
Be calm as thought and emotion come.
Breathe in open awareness.
Be undisturbed by thought.
Be undisturbed.
Continue energy breathing in open awareness.
Even with intense thoughts and emotions,

you can keep calm.
You can be fearless when labor comes.
You can bring calm into childbirth.
Breathe energy in open awareness.

All of life, all the universe, is present here and now.
Come into presence more and more.
Breathe in living presence.
Do this practice to prepare for childbirth.
When labor comes, you can do this practice.
You can remain undisturbed.
Remain undisturbed.
This is the way to calm birth.
When a contraction comes, breathe it in.
See and dispel fears that arise.
As the contraction fades return to energy breathing.
You're already doing it.
Relax and enjoy *Womb Breathing.*
It helps you stay calm in contractions.
Breathe calm between contractions.
Rest and breathe in awareness.
Breathe free.

This is a master path.
This is optimal breathing for childbirth,
full oxygenation and much more.
You're more alive in your breathing.
You're enjoying greater function.
Do something important for your child.
Do something important for your self.
Continue breathing into the Vase.

Giving and Receiving

The Potential of Healing in Childbirth

Introduction

The method of *Giving and Receiving*, innate to human capability, is designed to heal women of suffering in childbirth, and to help establish woman as healer and embodiment of wisdom to lift us into the great potential of human evolution.

In the history of the human species there have been many horrific events, but there has been no event more catastrophic than the murder of millions of women in Europe and America in the 16th and 17th centuries for the crime of practicing healing. It is the great potential of woman as healer and the great potential of human healing practices that set the stage for the healing of the damage done to womankind. It is the need to heal those wounds latent in women that makes today's need to heal and empower women in the process of childbirth an opportunity to bring light into the human species where darkness has prevailed too long.

The need to improve the prevailing childbirth practices and education is the opportunity to heal through new methods of childbirth preparation. And the immediate availability of the healing practice of *Giving and Receiving* is a method, placed in our hands by history, to heal what needs to be healed, in the greatest understanding of that need.

In the extraordinary tradition of the *Vajrayana* of Tibet, the Diamond Vehicle, it is understood that woman is the wisdom principle of the human species, as Ashley Montagu has importantly observed (1954). With appropriate methods in hand, now is the time for a dark part of history to be healed, and for womankind to heal the problems of childbirth—for the sake of the human species.

With the practice of *Giving and Receiving*, women first practice healing the damage to the psyche of womankind impacting childbirth today. Woman are able to sense and breathe in, take in, the energy caused by historical injustice, to take it into the light of their extended sense of body in childbirth, and to breathe out, radiate out into history all the healing energy needed to heal all that needs to be healed. The practice is done effortlessly, bountifully. The more women who do the practice to prepare for childbirth and the more they each do the practice, the more human history will be healed and the more woman as healer will arise through the process of childbirth. The intention to do so informs the energy of the practice.

It is evident from the work of pre- and perinatal psychology that the unnatural childbirth medicine prevalent the last few decades, involving ever more sophisticated kinds of drugs, anesthesia, and surgery, has caused unprecedented kinds of shock and trauma to babies and mothers. This has resulted in psychological and physiological imbalances that may begin to be healed through the far-reaching, innate capability that women can utilize as they prepare to conceive and give birth.

Giving and Receiving enables women to spontaneously engage and come into a new relationship with themselves and their history, to practice and cause the healing of their own birth experiences. The availability of the practice and the challenges of unnatural birth are the opportunity for women to arise as healers to practice the healing of their own birth experiences in preparation to give birth to a freer, healthier generation.

Preparing to give birth in this age of anxiety is an opportunity for women to practice the healing of their womb children, to free them from unprecedented disturbances coming into them from conception onward, to prevent disturbances and imbalances from affecting their development. *Giving and Receiving* is a method for prenatal fetal healing, nourishment, and support.

Giving and Receiving is an evolutionary practice of natural labor pain management. It works with *Womb Breathing* to help women use the experience of labor to empower themselves and others.

Description

Giving and Receiving can be practiced in any posture, at any time, but it's most effective to do this practice sitting. It's a method for healing in childbirth. A pregnant woman can practice *Giving and Receiving* for herself or for the child, or for both simultaneously. In this program it's used for prenatal care, for labor and delivery, and for postnatal care.

Please note that *Giving and Receiving* differs importantly from *Womb Breathing.* With *Womb Breathing* you take in vital energy from the air into your energy body. With *Giving and Receiving* you compassionately take in the energy of the suffering in yourself, in your child, or in someone else, and you see that energy dissolve into natural light in your body. You breathe out healing energy into yourself, your child, or someone else. *Womb Breathing* and *Giving and Receiving* must be practiced separately.

If a woman wants to prepare for conception and childbirth by healing her own adverse birth experiences and trauma, she can sit and follow the natural flow of her breath, easily and deeply. On her inhale she can breathe in the energy of any anxiety, suffering, any adverse condition she may have. What is inhaled dissolves into natural light in the body. She can breathe out into herself abundant healing energy. The breathing is not forced in any way. The breaths can be gentle and short, or longer and fuller, in the natural flow of the breath. The transition from inhale to exhale is effortless. The giving out of healing energy is bountiful, giving freely and graciously, generously, because the woman has come into her unlimited essential nature.

To do the practice for her child, the woman breathes in the energy of any difficulty that the child may have, however subtle it may be. She sees it dissolve into light in her body, and she breathes out healing energy into the child. What she intentionally takes in dissolves into live light in her cells, and she effortlessly breathes out healing energy.

A woman practicing *Giving and Receiving* during labor contractions inhales the pain of the contraction right into light in her body, and she exhales healing into birth. Her partner may also do this with her, for her and the child, experiencing the potential of bonding.

Commentary

This ancient wisdom method has been called "The Holy Secret" and "The Wish-Fulfilling Gem." Compassion is the wish-fulfilling gem. It's a Buddhist practice with important uses in medicine today. It's called *Ton Len* in Tibetan, which has been translated as "sending and receiving," or "exchanging oneself for another." It's a direct healing method that can be used to decrease anxiety and suffering and to reverse harmful conditions. *Giving and Receiving* helps women use their inherent healing skills. This method is a complement to most existing therapies and courses of treatment.

The basis of the practice is two-fold: compassion and the radiant energetic nature of the human body. The energy body is the source of inborn healing ability.

People on the birth team can do this practice to help the woman and child. They breathe in, taking in the energy of any illness, pain, or stress that the woman or womb child may have, and they breathe out, radiating healing energy into woman and child. If the birth is premature or if the child has problems, with *Giving and Receiving* anyone connected to the birth has a chance to help. The more time spent engaged in this practice, the more effective it will be. The pregnant woman practices healing herself and her child, entering her unlimited nature, bringing the practice and the experience of healing into birth. *Giving and Receiving* complements *Womb Breathing* during labor, facilitating breathing into contractions.

More about Breathing into Contractions

Though it's been demonstrated that women have innate ability to breathe into contractions, that doesn't imply that only the in-breath is important for doing that. *Giving and Receiving* is an inspired way to use both the inhale and the exhale, especially during long contractions when there may be a corresponding series of inhales and exhales. The exhales are important for the woman to breathe out healing energy into herself and to release pain and tension in the intensity of labor. Breathing into contractions as early as possible in labor enables women to gain psychological strength progressively throughout contractions, to recognize and dispel fears that arise, and to gain expanded health and power for herself, for her child, and for the species.

Key Points

- In this practice women connect with their innate healing ability, and they open to other dimensions of life in childbirth.
- It's healing to practice healing. The intention to heal oneself or another brings healing energy to the person who intends. Practicing healing is vital in childbirth.
- LIGHT IN THE BODY: The atomic mass of the human body is essentially electric light. Our atoms are made of electric charge and magnetic force. Electrons live and die in an instant, leaving brilliant traces of light. Light is our most core experience. To breathe the energy of suffering into body light we must breathe with compassion. In the practice of healing we learn to become living light.
- Research is exposing psychological and physiological trauma patterns and stress syndrome problems resulting from com-

mon OB practices, hence the escalating number of birth-related malpractice lawsuits. A primary use of *Giving and Receiving* is to help women heal any conditions that may reside in them, including obstetrically induced trauma, or birth-related physiological or psychological stress, in order to heal and resolve it, so as to not pass on the imprints of past negative birth experience to children.

- *Giving and Receiving* can be a vital complement to *Womb Breathing* during contractions. The use of *Giving and Receiving* throughout prenatal care develops an instinctive ability to take on one's pain and fear, one's challenges, to breathe them in and to breathe out the energy of support and healing into oneself, for the greater good. This is within every woman's capacity.
- *Giving and Receiving* is a supportive, nourishing practice that invites the father/partner to participate, honoring co-creation and co-healing.

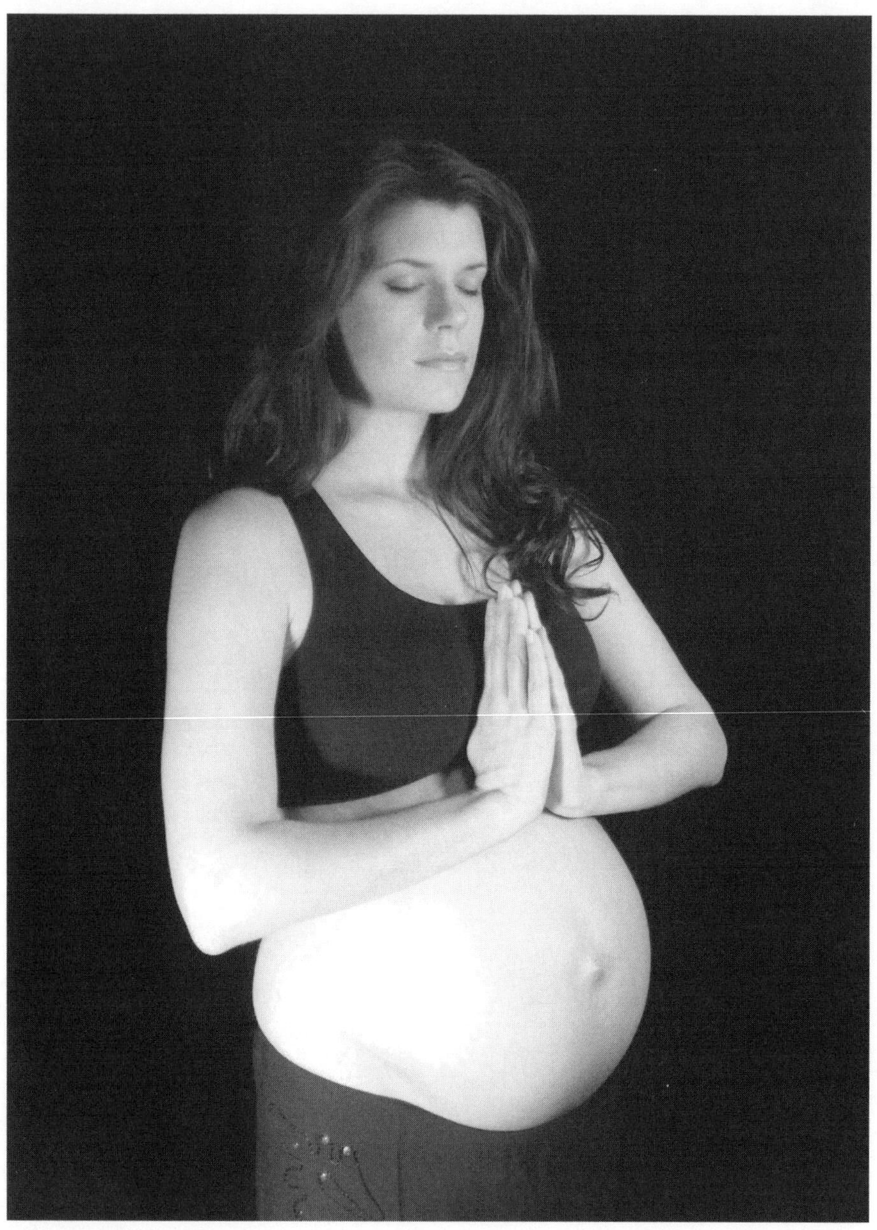

Giving and Receiving

(the practice)

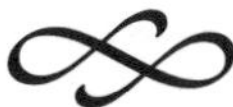

THE FOLLOWING IS A TRANSCRIPT of the audioguide transmission of this method. You can read this transcription and understand its intention. You can also obtain the audioguide CD and experience the method through audioguidance. If you are pregnant, the womb child will be responsive to the audioguidance.

Giving and Receiving is breathing healing.
It brings healing into childbirth.
Giving and Receiving is a famous practice from ancient wisdom applied to childbirth.
It's for whatever may need to be healed in the pregnant woman, her partner, and the child in the womb.

Sitting upright, balanced, at ease,
go with the natural flow of your breath.
Breathe in any health conditions you may have.
Let any harm or disturbance dissolve in light in your body.
Breathe out into your self all the healing energy you need.
Please practice this method of breathing.
On the in-breath, take in any disturbances there may be
in you, or in your child.
See the energy of any health challenge you may have
dissolve in light in your body.
With the out-breath, intend healing energies
into your self, or into the child, or into you both.
A child who is well
receives the energy as blessings.
Practice *Giving and Receiving* often.
Please do it now.

In the natural flow of your breath,
breathe in any tension or suffering that may be in you or in your child.
Take it to heart.
See that energy dissolve into light in your cells
and breathe out into your self and your child
all the healing energy you may need.
Breathe, healing yourself and your child.

Practice compassionate healing with your breath.
Compassionate breathing is empowering and far-reaching.
You can breathe into your own birth experience.
Any harm that may remain from your own birth
may be released by this practice now,
helping your child to be free.
What you breathe in from your birth dissolves in natural light in you.
Breathe out into your self and your child
all the healing energy you both may need.
It's time to heal with the breath.

Now turning toward another pregnant woman,
breathe into your body light any disturbance she may have.
You can do this easily, just as you did for your self and your child.
Whatever you breathe in dissolves in living light.
Effortlessly breathe out into that pregnant woman
all the healing energy she needs.
Please practice healing now.

There's no separation in the universal field.
You can reach any person directly in yourself,
wherever they are.
As you breathe in another woman's health challenges
you inseparably breathe in your own.
Breathe in easily, effortlessly giving that woman
your compassionate care.
All that you take in dissolves in light in you.
Breathe out, sending energies that nourish and heal.
Trust your ability to heal.

Now please turn your attention toward two or three pregnant women.

Effortlessly breathe their challenges into living light in your body.
Intend the energy of healing into those women.
Extend this practice of compassionate breathing now.
Please do it.

Taking this practice to a larger number of people,
think of a birthing center you know.
Imagine all the pregnant women, their partners,
the birthing personnel.
Go beyond what you think you can do.
Breathe in their discomfort, confusion, fear.
Let it all dissolve in the light in your body.
With clear intention, breathe out radiant healing energy
into all the people in the birthing center at once.
Give grace to the birthing center now.
You can do this.

When your labor contractions start,
you can breathe in the contraction.
You can breathe out opening.
If you practice now
you can prevent yourself from suffering.
You can breathe in the contraction.
You can breathe out release.
You can breathe grace into labor.
Please practice that now.

This is an ancient practice
proven effective through centuries of use.
Giving and Receiving can be done anywhere, anytime.
Be fearless in doing this compassionate breathing.
See that what you take in dissolves in light in you.
What you send out instantly connects.

The more you do this practice for yourself and your child,
the more effective it becomes.
The more you do this practice for others,
the more you heal your self and your child.
The more you do this practice the more life-giving you become.

This practice can be vital in postnatal care.
Please do this practice often.

Instinctive Movement and Vocalization in Labor

The Calm Birth methods, consistently practiced prenatally with steadfast intention to function at a higher evolutionary level during childbirth, provide a foundation for calm confidence. Labor and birth are eternal mysteries. No one can predict, control, or contain them. Birth is a mighty energy; women ride its waves with grace, open to its flow, or resist, vainly struggling against an irresistible power. The purpose of the Calm Birth program is to enable women to slow down and touch their inner core of being where the birth energy flows, enabling them to ride it with grace. The breathing practices, along with good childbirth education and exercises, prepare women to meet this primal force without fear, with faith in a good outcome, raising the quality of the birth whether it is natural or medicated.

In accord with the published findings of Michel Odent, M.D., and the perennial wisdom of midwives, the Calm Birth program affirms woman's need for privacy, low light, spontaneous movement, and freedom to vocalize undisturbed in labor. "—given the right kind of environment, where she could feel free and uninhibited—a woman could naturally reach a level of response [and resource] deeper within her than individuality, upbringing, or culture" (Odent, 1994, p. 13). In active labor, the Calm Birth breathing methods generally arise spontaneously as the woman instinctively returns to the freedom of open awareness, depending on the woman. Each labor is unique. How a woman has prepared and what kind of support she has in the moment will make a difference.

There is no doubt that free movement in labor is essential to natural birth, serving as entry to a more unlimited kind of being. Different kinds of positions, suggested by the sensations of contraction and cervical opening, enable the baby to more easily find her or his way and the mother to access a primal neural resource that knows how to lead her quickly and safely to birth. Laboring, pushing (if necessary), and giving birth from a standing or supported squatting position has been the choice of women for thousands of years. Waterbirth recognizes this ancient wisdom and takes it to a new evolutionary level. Warm water supports a woman's body and relaxes her, allowing her to birth vertically with minimum muscular tension.

Calm Birth is collecting data from midwives and doulas about remarkable movements they have witnessed arising spontaneously from laboring women. Some of these movements are becoming part of the training of Calm Birth teachers, to be used by birthing couples and their attendants as portals to profound somatic shifts, moving from the inside out during childbirth. A woman's own spontaneous movements are always preferred, but sometimes, when needed, a suggestion from another woman's birth experience can give rise to a sympathetic response.

Free vocalization in labor is an important sign of the progressive loss of inhibition that marks a woman's deepening into her core as she surrenders to and accesses the birth energy, sensing the power of her child's birth. The sound of personal power may arise: low primal growls, moans, sound song, and expressive yells often punctuate the natural flow of descent and opening. Sounds that spontaneously erupt are wonderful acts of release and augmentation of energy.

If loss of inhibition is slowed, birth attendants and partners may encourage the process by sounding or toning various syllables. As they calmly, deeply tone sounds, creating a sacred sound blanket around her, the woman may be inspired to join in. The sounds "ohhhhh," "ahhhhh," and "ouuuuu" help open the body. Just as the open mouth forms the sound, the cervix may open in response.

Seed syllable vocalization, in the lower registers, on the exhale of the breath, can help a woman stay relaxed and open and enter the inner sacred field. Different traditions use different syllables.

Energy centers of the body, called *chakras,* arranged vertically along the central energy channel, each have a characteristic sound syllable (seed syllable) that has been chanted for thousands of years for the opening and vitalization of that center. There is a collective global field that the laboring woman can access by sounding the syllable in a rhythmic pattern.

In one tradition, the first *chakra,* in the sacrum, corresponds to *Lam;* the second *chakra,* just above the pubic bones, is *Vam;* and the navel center is *Ram.* Normally, the first three *chakras* are the main energy centers involved in birth. Sounding these syllables in any way she wishes may serve a woman to access deep levels of instinctual wisdom and movement within herself. Concentrating her attention on the breath exhale and the sounding of the mantra syllable enables her to focus on energy release through sound, freeing her body to move with the birth energy as it opens to release her womb child. Even here, her previous practice of the Calm Birth methods nourishes her instinctual responses. All of the *chakras* may be actively involved in childbirth with the Calm Birth methods. Calm Birth recognizes that each woman will use the gifts she is inspired to use for her birth experience. Medicine woman knows her own best medicine.

Establishing an Effective Daily Practice

THE EFFECTIVENESS OF METHODS of new childbirth medicine, methods that women apply to empower themselves, depends on the quality of the application. Though critical mass is important—that is, the more the method is used the better—there are two factors that qualify that: the quality of attention and the energy of intention. They are closely related, but not the same.

In general, the stronger the intention to raise the quality of one's childbirth, the better the attention tends to be, and the more effective the practice. But it may be, for instance, that a woman has good quality attention to the methods for her first birth, and then finds that through developments in her being, when she applies the methods for the second, her intention is even stronger and the quality of her attention is even better. Or it can be that intention is strong, but individual life demands make attention difficult. Two factors can help in all cases: (1) raise the intention to benefit as many people as possible with your practice; (2) nurture your desire to raise the paradigm of childbirth science by establishing an effective daily practice.

In order to have calm breathing in labor, a daily practice of *Womb Breathing* is recommended. Women who establish a daily sitting practice develop biological enrichment and greater awareness. They intentionally give the child the biological benefits of prenatal care meditation, as previously described, and raise their level of awareness for making the right decisions during labor.

There may be nothing more important women can do to take charge of their health and their birthing process than to practice meditation every day. Daily morning practice is the best way to start the day to enrich pregnancy and for personal development.

It's important to practice every day if possible as a commitment to having a healthy pregnancy and birth. Practice as early in the morning as possible, to start the day in a healthy way. Find the quietest place available. Establish that place as your regular place of practice. If necessary it can be your bedroom. The more time you're able to commit to meditate for prenatal care and postnatal care the better. After giving birth, daily meditation practice is important for personal health and to raise the standard of childcare.

The Calm Birth training teaches women how to establish *Womb Breathing* before going to sleep in order to maintain the practice in lucid awareness while asleep. The body likes to do *Womb Breathing* on its own. By holding the intention before falling asleep, people can naturally perform the practice without conscious involvement. Remarkable benefits may come from a daily bedtime commitment.

Sustained practice is often empowering, and can be transformative. The healthful discipline of daily meditation practice is common ground for women who want to be teachers of childbirth meditation and who want to be a basis of a more enlightened society. The wider the scope of the intention of the practice the better. The best energy of intention is to want to fully benefit yourself, your child, your family, your society, and your planet by raising the quality of your childbirth. Also, as we have learned from advances of quantum physics (see Chapter VIII), whatever we do does not just happen locally; it also occurs universally, simultaneously. What we do to improve the quality of life on our planet affects all life, inseparably, everywhere in the universe. For optimal practice of new childbirth methods based on self-care, such as the Calm Birth methods, it's best to raise awareness and intention without limit.

VI

Eight Calm Births

Birth stories told by women who were active participants in giving birth often express a good deal of practical wisdom, inspiration, and information for other women. Positive stories shared by women who have had wonderful childbirth experiences are an irreplaceable way to transmit knowledge of a woman's true capacities in pregnancy and birth.

—Ina May Gaskin, *Ina May's Guide to Childbirth*

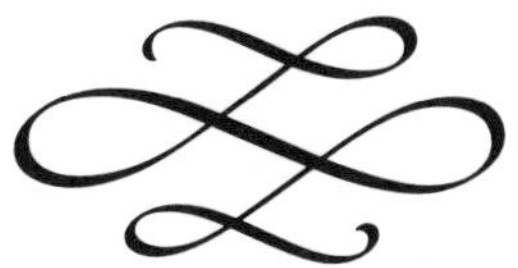

The Calm Birth Program

The Calm Birth program was presented in Southern Oregon hospitals starting in 1998: Rogue Valley Medical Center (RVMC), Medford; Providence Medford Medical Center (PMMC); and Ashland Community Hospital (ACH). In October 1999, the Calm Birth methods were presented at RVMC for the combined OB/GYN departments of RVMC and PMMC. Six-hour training seminars have been presented at each of the above facilities, and a weekly class has been offered at ACH. From 1999 to the present, the California Board of Nursing has given education credits to people who attend the trainings.

Following is a selection of interviews with eight women and their partners of the more than nine hundred couples who have given birth using the Calm Birth methods. The interviews are postnatal unless otherwise indicated. It is a record of applied childbirth meditation. In it are descriptions of new childbirth experience based on new childbirth methods.

Gahl Moriel

Ellen had two sons and she became pregnant again at the age of forty-two. Her husband, Douglas, is a respected doctor. From early in the pregnancy Ellen fully applied the Calm Birth methods, wanting a natural childbirth. The pregnancy proceeded beyond the due date, and Ellen continued the Calm Birth practices sensing a special opportunity for communion with the child. Three weeks beyond the due date she was able to continue *Womb Breathing* throughout labor. Afterward she said, "Deep breathing was natural and helped the birth process flow forward." She gave birth to a baby girl. Immediately after the delivery the wide-eyed child made eye contact with Ellen, and then rested peacefully on her breast.

Parents: Ellen and Douglas
Baby: Gahl Moriel
Birth date: August 7, 2003
Birth weight: 8 lbs 15 oz
Interviewer: Robert Newman
Interview date: July 18, 2003 (prenatal)

Prenatal Interview with Ellen

CB: The first thing that you mentioned that you wanted was calm, compared to what you experienced in your first two births. Do you remember when you were introduced to the Calm Birth methods?

Ellen: About four months ago I received the CD of the Calm Birth methods.

CB: Concerning the *Practice of Opening,* how often have you been doing that?

Ellen: I've been pretty consistent. It's been about three or four times a week. I've been practicing the whole CD, all three methods. I've mostly been using the CD to practice the methods because that way I can focus the best. The texts [of the methods] are really interesting.

CB: In terms of where the language of the methods brings you, what it facilitates for you, are you experiencing greater union in bonding with the child than in your previous births?

Ellen: I don't think so. It's been more my relationship with myself that's been changed—the understanding of my own empowerment—how to be more available to myself. Now I can understand what I'm thinking; I can notice what I'm thinking and where that's leading me. And then I come back to the methods and have thoughts that are more conducive to a calm birth.

CB: We've been told by people using the *Practice of Opening* for the birth that in so many ways it brings you into the life force in your cells, life force on a cellular level. Women say that the practice brings you to your life force in an empowering way. Do you think that the completeness of going through your body, system after system, coming into the life force—have you had that experience? Does that have something to do with what you called "empowerment" in this practice?

Ellen: Absolutely. It's been very helpful. It gives me something solid to come back to. Now my body has been trained to get into that relaxation space. I think the baby definitely responds to that, understands that, knows that. In that way the relationship has been deepened. I've always been very close with my babies.

CB: Has the practice brought you a deeper knowledge of your body and its systems, in making you feel stronger?

Ellen: Yes.

CB: Is part of what's making you feel stronger, knowledge of your capabilities?

Ellen: Yes, and to be able to go to that place, to go to those experiences and access the energy.

CB: So the practice gives you energy, and would you say it gives you a deeper sense of your own capability, a deeper confidence in your capability, going into all those systems and feeling them empowering you?

Ellen: Yes. I think the experience of feeling more alive is in itself empowering.

CB: How often have you been doing the practice of *Womb Breathing,* as far as listening to the audioguide?

Ellen: The same as the *Practice of Opening,* at least three or four times a week. And then whenever I'm sitting down I remember; my body remembers the practice and does it.

CB: That's the big difference between these two practices. In the *Practice of Opening* you have to lie down and follow the audioguide through the whole practice. With *Womb Breathing,* it gives you the instruction to enable you to do the practice any time, as much as possible. Even at night, in your sleep. That's why *Womb Breathing* is the main practice coming into labor. So you've done it every day then?

Ellen: Oh, yes. At least several times a day, I'll sit down to read a book to my kids, and as soon as I sit I remember to do the practice.

CB: Mind/body medicine has extended the way the human body is seen. It's seen as an energy body now, with energy systems. Doctors are using that knowledge more in understanding what the body is. It's being taught more in medical schools. In the *Womb*

Breathing practice you're trained to breathe vital energy in the air into your energy body systems. This extends childbirth anatomy. How has the practice of *Womb Breathing* extended your sense of your body? Like when you breathe into the Vase?

Ellen: Yes, like a vessel. My understanding of it is that it's more visceral. It's not a head thing.

CB: You understand that the Life Vase you breathe into is not the same as the womb. The Vase is a part of the energy body very near the womb. You're breathing vital essence toward the unborn baby when you breathe into the Life Vase. But it's not breathing into the womb even though the practice is called *Womb Breathing*. Is that clear to you?

Ellen: Yes. It's breathing into the *Hara* [the "vital center"].

CB: And that's working for you?

Ellen: I believe it because I do feel something; so the baby must feel it. I know that the baby feels whatever I feel. So if I'm enriching myself the baby is getting that.

CB: You said that when you sit and read to the children the *Womb Breathing* comes back to you. It was our intention that the *Womb Breathing* would become a natural ongoing process. Then when you get to labor, when you start to get distracted by contractions, involuntarily your body starts to do the practice. All the women who have used our methods in labor have said that *Womb Breathing* came to them throughout labor. Their body would do it. The body likes to do it.

Ellen: Right. That's great.

CB: Can you say that in some sense the *Womb Breathing* practice has transformed your sense of body and breathing?

Ellen: Yes. I think that whenever I've done the practice consistently it's transformed me. It's always a positive experience. I always feel relaxed and more in touch with myself and the baby.

CB: This is a practice that comes from ancient wisdom. Masters have used this method for centuries, the breathing of vital essence from the air into the *Hara*, the vital center, the Life Vase. In terms of the sacredness of life it's supposed to give you greater respect for what the air is, what we usually take for granted, and this practice brings a greater respect for the body. Is that true for you?

Ellen: Yes, I think it's definitely amazing. It's a miracle what exactly can transpire. I take breathing for granted; but to really focus on it, to be under the practice, under the influence of the practice, what can happen is not an ordinary thing.

CB: Please say again how you're using the word "miracle" there.

Ellen: I think any time I step out of my ordinary unconscious state it's a miracle. And to actually slow down and do the practice and experience it is calling in another energy. It kind of pushes me to another level of waking up. Therefore, I appreciate my life, and life itself; I feel more alive. I'm more connected with the baby, more connected with everyone and everything.

CB: Would you say that *Womb Breathing* builds on your experience of the *Practice of Opening* in giving you greater knowledge of your body and a more empowered sense of your own capability?

Ellen: Yes. I feel that *Opening* is the framework, the groundwork, and the two practices, *Womb Breathing* and *Giving and Receiving*, are a way to create it as a living thing, as something that's more accessible.... *Giving and Receiving* is interesting. I take some prenatal yoga classes. And I find myself thinking about the *Giving and Receiving* practice in those classes, when I'm with other pregnant women in the class, or when we run into each other in town. Some of them have issues.

CB: You mean conditions they have to deal with?

Ellen: Yes. And to be able to send them this—to give to them, to take in something and turn it into light—I think that's really good.

CB: *Giving and Receiving* is a famous healing practice from ancient wisdom. There've been amazing success stories with the practice (Sogyal, 1994). For the use of it in childbirth, does it add to the sense of empowerment you have in the other practices?

Ellen: I think the practice is really connected with people, feeling good intention, praying for them to resolve whatever their obstacles are.

Cooper William

MOLLY HAD A PHYSICAL PROBLEM that made intensive medical care necessary during her first childbirth. That resulted in having the birth pushed with pitocin, which then resulted in an epidural block. Molly felt this had been unnecessary, and she regretted not having the birth experience she had hoped for. There was no physical pain but there were lingering unresolved feelings. For her second pregnancy, four years later, she was determined to eliminate medical interventions as much as possible. She had learned meditation as a child, and when her mother recommended the Calm Birth methods early in the pregnancy, Molly eagerly applied them and was able to experience an empowered birth.

Parents: Chris and Molly
Baby: Cooper William
Birth date: March 23, 2002
Birth weight: 8 lbs 9 oz
Interviewer: Whitney Wolf
Interview date: May 21, 2002

Postnatal Interview with Molly

CB: What is your memory of the first time you were introduced to the Calm Birth childbirth methods?

Molly: My mother introduced the methods to me. She sent me the audioguide and an article about Calm Birth. I remember listening to the audio and thinking that some of it was things I already knew how to do like relaxing from your toes all the way up to your head. And just thinking that it was a really interesting thing to try.

CB: How far along in your pregnancy were you when you began using the Calm Birth childbirth methods?

Molly: Maybe two months.

CB: What kind of previous meditation training have you done?

Molly: I had been taught how to meditate as a small child and would sort of practice it on and off as an adult. I'd learned different kinds of relaxation techniques.

CB: What was it you were looking for and wanted to find when you were introduced to the Calm Birth childbirth methods?

Molly: I was just looking for anything that might help the labor process, tools to use that let me feel like I had something to be proactive with, in having a better attitude about the birth, more knowledge to feel more confident.

CB: Did you experience it that way?

Molly: Yes, I did. I felt like I had more of an understanding of and an appreciation of the labor process instead of it being just something hard that you go through. It's a simple part of the process that brings the baby to you. And then I felt that I was more confident because I had some extra tools.

CB: How would you describe the tools you learned from the Calm Birth childbirth methods?

Molly: The ability to focus and the breathing was really helpful. The visualizing was very helpful and some of the words I remembered from the audiocassette. Like the fact that the contractions are bringing the baby to you, so it is helpful to work with them, not against them. Also relaxing your whole body while in the middle of the pain.

CB: How often do you recall doing the *Practice of Opening* before you gave birth?

Molly: It was sporadic, not really a regular thing. Sometimes it would be a couple of times per week, sometimes more.

CB: Usually in the evening?

Molly: Yes, usually in the evening right before going to bed.

CB: And how about the practice of *Womb Breathing*?

Molly: It was about the same. I would do whichever side of the audiocassette was ready to go, instead of rewinding it, so I'd alternate the methods. Sometimes I'd do the breathing for relaxation on my own without the tape. During pregnancy I woke up a lot during the night to go to the bathroom or because I was uncomfortable or something. I'd have a hard time going back to sleep so I'd do the practice on my own to relax.

CB: So it appears that you could recall the Calm Birth methods after you'd done them a while?

Molly: Yes.

CB: Were you able to recall the methods during the time that you were at the hospital?

Molly: Yes, I brought the audiocassette with the audio player with me to the hospital and during the first few hours I wore the headphones, playing the audiocassette until things became more intense. Then I would sit in the rocking chair doing the breathing on my own.

CB: Was *Womb Breathing* helpful for your ability to recognize the difference between pain and suffering? In labor it's pretty normal to have pain or discomfort, but we can get caught in identifying with the pain and it becomes suffering. Were you able to recognize the difference between the pain and the suffering using *Womb Breathing*?

Molly: Toward the end I didn't because I was having a really hard time, right before I decided to have an epidural. I was having heavy contractions and screaming a lot. But I thought to myself that *Womb Breathing* was a way of going with it so I was doing that to open up to the process. And then the contractions would be over and I would cry. It was really interesting to me. I was doing a lot of self-talk like "okay, this is hard and it's painful, but just go with whatever you're feeling instead of being stronger than you are. Go where the emotion is taking you." This self-talk and awareness really helped me. Yes, this is painful and I am going to express that. With my daughter's birth I was given pitocin and an epidural, which was okay, and I just hung out till it was time to push and everything was kind of mellow and easy. But this time it was different. This time I really wanted to experience the true sense of labor, to see what that feels like.

CB: It sounds as though you were actively participating rather than watching it from afar.

Molly: Yes, exactly. And that's what I wanted. I wanted to try all of the things that you read about, standing, sitting, rocking in a chair, my husband right there with me so that we were there doing it together.

CB: As a result of your commitment to using the Calm Birth methods what stands out to you as being different between the first and second childbirth experiences?

Molly: With my first child I guess I was not with the experience, and with my second child I was with the experience. The Calm Birth methods helped me with my anxiety levels and the ability to relax. The methods also helped me with some of the sleep problems that I had. And as I mentioned before, I felt more in control of the labor process. I had more information and more resources. That was the biggest thing I think.

CB: Would you say that the Calm Birth methods helped you in any way to experience a calmer childbirth?

Molly: Yes. Yes. I mean you know that the labor process is an intense painful thing and I don't think that you can really get away from that. But while I was in the middle of it I was feeling like this was what I really wanted to do, experience childbirth. Childbirth was a positive experience because I had some information from the Calm Birth audiocassettes that was helpful and I felt more confident in what I was doing and in how I was doing it. I was more in control.

CB: How did you feel more confident? What do you think was giving you the confidence?

Molly: I guess because I'd practiced the Calm Birth audioguides I knew that I could get myself relaxed. I knew that I could do the *Womb Breathing* and that would help me. And it did! It doesn't take the pain away, of course, but I just felt like I was a little more able to handle it. It wasn't as scary. It wasn't as unmanageable.

CB: Do you see benefits of the Calm Birth methods in Cooper?

Molly: I think that he's calm in one sense in that he doesn't cry a lot and it is fairly easy to figure out what he needs.... He hardly cries. He sleeps really well at night and he likes to giggle and move around.

CB: So as far as what was happening and what you were doing, were you aware of any synchronizing of the movements between you and Cooper during the contractions and delivery? Was there any kind of dialogue that you were aware of?

Molly: I remember the nurse was telling me that they showed me on the monitor where he was moving down. Then I thought okay, along with my visualization of the contractions moving him down I'm also going to open up to let him come out. It wasn't obvious that I was talking with him or doing visualization with him, but I was trying to have this flow going between us and that is how I visualized it, that he was like a river.

CB: When the contractions were coming and caused your body to get tight, were you able to return to your *Womb Breathing*?

Molly: Yes. I would notice the contraction would come and I could see the baby on the monitor coming and I could feel him so I would start to tense up and then I'd start breathing, breathing really deeply, and I'd close my eyes sometimes or sometimes I'd look and focus on something else, or get my husband. I'd make a point of opening up and releasing him instead of tightening up more.

CB: Was *Womb Breathing* helpful for you to stay with those hours of labor and to stay with it with greater awareness and ability?

Molly: Yes. *Womb Breathing* was a big part. I noticed that since I learned how to breathe more deeply, I instantly felt better.

CB: Please speak about breathing vital energy in the air. How was that helpful while you were doing *Womb Breathing?*

Molly: That was helpful in the sense that it was a visualization for me. As I was breathing I visualized light coming into me and going down to him [Cooper, the baby].

CB: How did the visualization affect your experience through contractions and delivery?

Molly: Well, it helped me by counteracting the pain.

CB: Like an antidote?

Molly: With pain there is a tendency of saying "pain is bad; this is bad because it hurts." This translates into something negative. Then doing *Womb Breathing* helped me to say I am bringing in what he and I both need to do, this movement to open up and to relax. This is part of what we need for him to come out.

CB: The first few hours of labor were you able to return to *Womb Breathing?*

Molly: Yes. Maybe the first six or so hours, and then the last hour I wasn't really able to do that. I got so tired.

CB: How were the Calm Birth methods helpful for you to calm and to listen to your own impulses for movement?

Molly: I think the methods helped me stay in touch with my body and to listen to it, moving with the process rather than fighting it.

CB: During pregnancy was there any kind of movement rhythm that you experienced with the baby?

Molly: Yes, the rhythm in movement with the Calm Birth methods helped me to relax and synchronize with the baby before birth.

It also helped to reduce anxiety and hold a focus.

CB: Was *Womb Breathing* supportive in the natural movement for you during childbirth?

Molly: Yes. With *Womb Breathing* if you're breathing deeply you can't be tensed up in your body. If you're really doing *Womb Breathing* it helps you to relax, helping everything open and release.

CB: Did the Calm Birth methods give you a sense of self-empowerment during childbirth in the hospital?

Molly: Yes. I felt like I had more tools to use and something to actually practice so I could be more proactive and leading the process of childbirth instead of being led by the process. I felt more confident like I could handle it and I knew what to do.

CB: What positive benefits do you see in your child from exercising the Calm Birth childbirth methods during pregnancy, contractions, and delivery?

Molly: I didn't notice so much with him during my pregnancy. I noticed more with me. I was able to be more relaxed, less anxious, and sleep better. I also believe that the Calm Birth methods helped the process move forward more easily.

CB: Are you referring to the contractions?

Molly: Yes. *Womb Breathing* helped me to work with the process instead of fighting it. This helped me a lot.... I believe the labor would have gone on longer if I didn't do *Womb Breathing.* He [Cooper] is a mellow baby.... He doesn't cry very much and I think that's a benefit from Calm Birth.

CB: In seeing the positive benefits of the Calm Birth practices in your child, how does that make you feel about yourself?

Molly: I feel really good about myself and I enjoyed doing it. Calm Birth was helpful for me and I think it was helpful for Cooper too. Calm Birth was something that I could do that was noninvasive, you know, empowering. I could be in control and choose how to do it, use it how I wanted to use it.

CB: What positive benefits do you see in yourself by using the Calm Birth practices?

Molly: I feel healthy and empowered.

CB: How do you feel healthy?

Molly: The *Womb Breathing* helps me to relax because I tend to have anxiety problems and stress. The Calm Birth methods do a lot to keep this sort of thing in check and I feel better, less stressful with more energy, able to handle stress better.

CB: What can you say about the methods and the sense of safety you experienced?

Molly: I didn't feel the childbirth experience was something negative. I always thought it was a positive thing. Calm Birth helped me to be proactive in the labor and in the pregnancy.

CB: Can you sense that your prenatal Calm Birth efforts have given you and your child benefits that are long term?

Molly: I know that for me there will be long-term benefits and I can assume that for Cooper there will be too. We will see how he develops. I feel I have the Calm Birth methods forever.

CB: When you hold and feed Cooper, do you ever notice your body returning to the calming method?

Molly: Yes. I do the breathing.

CB: What do you notice in Cooper when you do these methods?

Molly: He will calm down because sometimes he gets kind of frantic and now he's making eye contact with me during nursing, which is very nice.

Hana Leigh

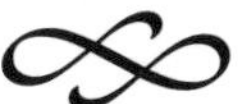

LATE IN HER THIRD PREGNANCY, Clee expressed interest in meditation to a midwife she had just chosen to help her with her birth, which she wanted to be completely natural. The midwife was trained in the Calm Birth methods, and recommended that Clee get in touch with the Calm Birth program. The result was that even though Clee received the methods only eight days before the birth, the following account of the birth testifies to the fact that even if a woman is introduced to the Calm Birth methods toward the end of the pregnancy, the methods can be transformative.

Parents: Clee and Austen
Baby: Hana Leigh
Birth date: February 26, 2001
Birth weight: 7 lbs 4 oz
Interviewer: Whitney Wolf
Interview date: May 25, 2001

Postnatal Interview with Clee and Austen

CB: Hana Leigh was born on February 26, 2001, eight days after you were introduced to the Calm Birth methods. What were your first experiences, once you received the Calm Birth instructions?

Clee: Just taking the time to sit, to be centered, and go inward and to check in. That quiet space. It really helped a lot.

CB: How did you find taking that inward space helpful at that point in your pregnancy?

Clee: It helped to reduce stress and clarify some things within myself. It provided me a calm space. It definitely helped me to calm down and feel more centered and balanced, and ready to deal with the next day, with my other children, and all the input and stimulation of the day.

CB: How would you describe your experience?

Clee: Definitely a sense of being more centered, calm, and present. I was able to stay that way even with a lot of things that were going on. During the birth I was able to be in the present moment, with the pain, not wondering what it would be in an hour from now, or going away from the moment. It really helped me to be fully in the birth experience.

CB: Austen, did you have any kind of experience where you could imagine the womb in yourself with the child in your womb?

Austen: Yes, definitely. I had a couple of dreams that were very lucid where I felt that I was pregnant and I could feel Hana Leigh was really active in my belly. She was moving around. Actually I think what happened is that I fell asleep with my hand on Clee's belly and she was moving all around when I fell into a dream space with that happening. And then I had this dream that she was in my tummy moving all around and I think that in the real space my hand was still on Clee's belly. I remember doing the meditation and I felt a sense of warm energy in my tummy and allowing this.

CB: Could you actually be present with the experience of being in union with the pregnancy?

Austen: Yes. The sense of breathing to nourish your baby felt really good and I could connect with that. The *Womb Breathing* actually helped me to remember to breathe to nourish my own inner baby. It was great.

Clee: Yes, it was nice to share that experience together.

CB: By having the Calm Birth methods, how did this pregnancy differ from your previous pregnancies?

Clee: This time in the actual labor I was able to be more in the moment, breathing and opening up to that pain, not resisting it as I had done before. I attribute that to a lot of things, but it helped me by listening to the tape and practicing—being more aware and in the moment and more able to open up to that pain rather than resisting it.

CB: How did the Calm Birth methods help you with the pain by being present with it and not resisting it?

Clee: Being present with the pain and not resisting it was amazing. It was the most powerful, wonderful experience. It was a journey and a great adventure rather than a scary drawn-out nightmare.

CB: The pain and the fear appear to be connected. If you resist the pain it leads to more fear. If you surrender and open, the fear and resistance seem to resolve themselves.

Clee: Exactly. Because being in the moment you are just being there, fully feeling. You are open and just there. Fear for me comes when you're worrying what is going to happen, the next contraction, or when the baby comes, grasping for a moment that isn't real. Then you are missing out on being in the moment, not being able to be open, because you are resisting something that has not even happened. It is kind of hard to explain; I would say that the pain didn't feel as painful.

CB: Austen, in the time that you came into contact with the Calm Birth methods and doing the *Womb Breathing* with Clee, was there any kind of shift of function or awareness for you?

Austen: It definitely helped me with a sense of connection. It helped shift me into a balanced perspective. Whereas before, being a father in a pregnancy you are feeling a sense of more like "I am going to take care of the other duties. I am not really in charge of nourishing the baby in the body besides cooking meals for the mama." It reminded me, it might have been something that I read or heard on the Calm Birth audio, that the father is important, spiritually and energetically nourishing the baby with his thoughts and energy. So there is a real connection. It definitely helped me to see that.... After receiving the Calm Birth methods and before she was born, it was really rich with magical experiences. Probably dreams too, but it's hard to remember.

Clee: That's because it was like a kind of dreamy space around the birth.

Austen: We talked about it being only a week and two days that we had the tapes, but when Clee first heard from Rhione, the midwife, about this opportunity, that someone was writing a book and was offering classes and the tape, that was sort of like an initial connection with the Calm Birth program. That was the first time I'd really heard of anything about pregnant women or couples meditating to alleviate the fears and discomforts in labor. I'd never heard anything about that. That was the first connection. And that was a couple of weeks prior to when Clee met you and received the methods.

Clee: The day before the birth I came outside and hung out. We had a beautiful, wonderful day. I was having light cramping. Went to bed that night and woke up about three in the morning. What I recall is Anaya [their two-year-old son] screaming "baby!" in the middle of the night and waking me up. That is what I recall. I recall him saying "BABY." Austen doesn't remember hearing him say that, but that is what I heard and it was like I was in labor!

CB: That's beautiful! A Near Birth Experience through the family system.

Clee: Right. It was pretty amazing. And I woke up and said, "I'm in labor." And I got up and I was in labor for sure.... Then I said that I was cold so we made the house really warm. The midwives said, "I think that you might be in labor." I asked Austen to time the contractions. I thought the baby was going to come relatively quickly. So, I was really able to be present, to really open up to the pain.

CB: I know that when we first met, you shared with me that you wanted to really come to a place where you could open and surrender.

Clee: That was my big hope for my experience with labor and I was really able to do that and it was so great. Then Austen called the midwives at some point. I was able to go through labor by myself for a while. They got here just as the sun was rising.

Austen: They got here right when the light was coming in. It was amazing. They had just walked in. We had had some worries that Anaya and Kai' [their sons] would be upset and be awake and want lots of attention. But they were sound asleep and they slept through the majority of it.

Clee: Anaya woke up about an hour before the birth.... I went on amazing journeys. I just went into myself and it was like I was feeling myself like you were talking about in the meditation tape [Calm Birth audioguide] how you can get way out there and the voice brings me back; I was able to bring myself back. I would get real involved in the pain and then I would feel okay, and then I would imagine whales under water giving birth and I would think, wow, you know I can do this. And then I thought about all of the women that were giving birth in that moment and all those who have given birth. I was really able to ground myself in these real feelings of power and the beauty of it, rather than feeling I can't do this because it's such a hard thing. I am doing this! There are hundreds of women doing this right now. I can do this! I am doing it!... The midwives came in and we were sitting there. I was able to let them touch my body and open up to their love, and the same with Austen, without feeling resistance. Then the contractions started getting really strong and the pain was getting more and more difficult for me to handle. I said that I wanted to get into the water and I got in the water. Not too long after I got in the water, maybe an hour, she was born.

Austen: Just as the sun was rising—I remember them saying, "Oh, I see her head," and I was holding Anaya and walking around. Maybe it was ten minutes before she was born that the sun peaked—there is a ridge on the east side—and there was this glimmer of sun peaking over that ridge.

Clee: I was really calm. I remembered the pushing part in the last intense part of labor was like screaming for me my last two childbirths. This time I was able to use my voice and make these real guttural songs [she expressed her sounds as she explained what she was experiencing].

Austen: Yes. I've heard these sounds in songs before in Tibetan chants sung by monks that are real deep. That's what she sounded like when she was in the water.

Clee: It was awesome.

CB: Have you ever experienced these sounds in yourself before?

Clee: Not in myself. No. It felt so good. I felt so grounded and rooted in strength, like ah—the earth. I really don't have words for it, but it really helped me. It was a tool for using my voice like I had been wanting to do in my previous births without screaming or distress.

CB: Were you aware of your breathing during the contractions, or in delivery, by returning to *Womb Breathing?*

Clee: Oh, yes. I was very conscious of my breath throughout, the whole way. While I was going on a journey inside myself, the breath was the physical manifestation of the other part that was helping me remain open. Helping me to be flexible and open. It was the breath.

CB: When the contractions relaxed, did you find yourself doing the *Womb Breathing?*

Clee: Yes. Right in between while I was awaiting the next contraction and I was taking time to breathe and center myself.

Austen: And she was subconsciously doing *Womb Breathing*. Her body reverted to that naturally.

Clee: Definitely. Yes. It was really great. It was beautiful. It was wonderful. It went really smoothly. It was really calm. She came out and she was just sitting there and I rubbed her back and it was really peaceful space for her to come into. Everything had been peaceful.

Austen: The midwives commented that it was hard for them to leave this house.

CB: How was it hard for them to leave?

Austen: Because it was being in life itself. Sometimes you know the labor gets intense and people are all involved and there is lots of tension and the woman is in a lot of pain rather than letting it just flow. Clee was really able to handle the intensity of energy [Clee comments with "yes"], to be able to handle it and harness it rather than fight it because it is literally like the universe pouring through the mother giving birth. That energy is coming through. Clee was to let the energy flow rather than be afraid of it.

CB: Do you think that Clee was able to engage the labor and delivery through her breath and affect everyone else around her?

Austen: Yes. Yes. Definitely. At one point one of the midwives commented that she has been doing childbirth for a long time and it was a great day for other women across the world giving birth because they could tap into that energy that Clee was experiencing.

Clee: Every step of the way, the first thing I would do was check in with her [Hana Leigh] and recognize that this pain is bringing my baby closer to me. I don't know other than I was just opening up to her coming through. It was like I was in a process of birth. I felt like that is how I had to prepare myself to be her mother and to know her.

CB: I'm interested to know if was there a need to push?

Clee: I did go through a little bit of wanting to bear down and push as hard as I could, and I did that push, push, push. It was really hard. Then the attending midwives reminded me saying, "Open yourself up and allow the baby to come through and be with your breath." Then I was able to let her come through more naturally rather than trying to push. I experienced both sides of what you are saying: feeling the desire to get the pain over with, and the releasing through my breath.

CB: What do you feel was the urge to want to push?

Clee: I was ready for her to come out. I want to see you now you're so close. And then wanting to be in control of it, wanting to be active in it rather than opening up and being responsible with this energy.

CB: Impatient with the timing—

Austen: Yeah, wanting to have a sense of control.

CB: What was the difference when you were pushing versus when you felt that you were being moved?

Clee: When I was trying to push, there was a sense of forceful energy trying to get something out. She was resisting it.

CB: How did you know that?

Clee: It was a feeling that she would come down and slip back up and I could feel her doing it. There was a sense of trying to make something happen while not really knowing if it's not going to happen. If you just keep pushing, pushing, pushing, pushing, it's resistance.

CB: Would you say that the Calm Birth methods were helpful for you, Clee, to calm down and listen to your inner impulses of movement?

Clee: Yes, definitely. Every time I did it, several times before the birth, it was very helpful. I can imagine had I implemented it much earlier it could have been more helpful. Taking the time to do that for myself, to listen to the tape and do the practice, that's a key. I think women would really benefit from that, taking the time and space to breathe and go within.

CB: Do you feel that you accomplished what your intention was when we first met when you expressed to me what your concerns were and what you wanted to accomplish with this labor and delivery with Hana Leigh?

Clee: Oh, yes. I was definitely able to do what I wanted to, which was to open up and allow the universe of life to be poured through me and be able to embrace it and enjoy it and see it as a real gift. When you fully open up to it, it's this amazing, strong, powerful *love* flowing through you! It's really an amazing gift! [Clee's voice as she was expressing her experience here became very enlivened, rich with tones.]

CB: I can feel it right now with you voicing it. The power went right through me, the power again, how beautiful.

Clee: It is and I feel blessed to have been able to get to a space to feel it, instead of resisting it and being afraid of it because it's really powerful.

McKane Scott

TAMARA AND DAVID, a young couple remarkable for their physical beauty and intelligence, came to the Calm Birth program early in their first pregnancy. They applied the practices earnestly, desiring a natural childbirth. Unfortunately an OB nurse at the hospital misjudged the position of the baby in the uterus, not understanding that it was breech, and encouraged premature pushing during labor. This resulted in various difficulties and ended in a C-section delivery. However, Tamara was able to maintain an exceptional calm and clarity, which benefited all concerned. As the following description relates, she considered it an empowered birth. The child emerged calm and aware.

Parents: Tamara and David
Baby: McKane Scott (Mickey)
Birth date: October 10, 1998
Birth weight: 8 lbs 8 oz
Interviewer: Whitney Wolf
Interview date: April 15, 2000

Postnatal Interview with Tamara and David

Tamara: Telling the story, basically my water broke, and I realized I was going into labor. And it was my first time. I was thinking, I'm going to have this period where the contractions are going to be really slow and calm and I'm going to play the Calm Birth tape, and listen to it. As soon as my water broke I was pacing the house. Altered. My contractions were really intense. I was told afterward it was just because of the breech position. He was against my pelvis. So I labored for eighteen hours. No drugs. Thank God I had Dave and my other two birth coaches breathing in my face telling me not to push. That was another thing. I wanted to push because of the position for a lot longer than most people do. And then I ended up having a C-section.

CB: Did they attempt to turn the baby at all?

David: I think they didn't diagnose his position—

Tamara: Until much later I think. I didn't have a chance to meditate. As I said, as soon as my water broke I was pacing and basically I walked up and down that hospital the whole eighteen hours. I couldn't sit. But I think the part that helped me was to stay in control. To know that I could breathe into the pain, not let the pain take over my body, freak me out, and feel out of control. And, now that I think about it, the Calm Birth methods were very helpful. A lot of women if it's their first time won't know what they're going to experience. Nothing prepares you. You get fight-or-flight and you're thinking, Okay, here we go. I don't know. Dave, you think I remained pretty calm? Despite the positioning?

David: Yeah, I think you were great. It was extremely valuable information and entirely positive in all respects. We were 100 percent committed to the Calm Birth methods.

Tamara: Yes.

David: You incorporated it partly into how you went through the birth. We weren't talking about Calm Birth while we were going through it, but it was in our psyche somewhere.

Tamara: In our systems.

CB: What was your first impression of the Calm Birth class, do you remember?

Tamara: Yeah. I felt empowered. I thought this is great, this information. That was the first class we ever took.

CB: Did you attend with her, David?

David: Yes.

Tamara: So I think that was my main feeling—of control, that I don't have to give my power away to the doctor, which I think I normally would have. If I didn't have the Calm Birth training I would have been so freaked out like this is my first time, and I would have given them more power than was necessary. So that part really helped me. That was my first impression of the class, about empowerment. Karen, my doctor, afterward came up to me and said, you know, I just want to say how impressed [I was] with how awake and aware you were. It made her feel comfortable. She knew that I wanted a vaginal delivery. I think she felt bad that didn't happen.

CB: So being aware and present doesn't mean we always control everything.

Tamara: Exactly, that's true. That's a lesson of life for sure.

CB: But you can be present and aware of your steps. That's a wonderful thing to be given from the Calm Birth methods. That's really the intention of Calm Birth, to open into greater awareness and to be present. It sounds like you've really received that intention. There's still something that's resonating.

David: Absolutely. Tamara's personality and the way she does things is not calm, meditative. She usually steps up to a challenge more in an intense manner. Which I mean, you can do, I think, at that level of meditation. As I said, I think you can be in a meditative state to a certain extent while you're going through this far more physical activity.

Tamara: Exactly, and I feel like I was. I didn't feel so out of it. I was directing these guys to breathe with me.

David: There was no screaming or hysterics. Everything was very calm the whole time, but she had to stay active, on the move.

Tamara: Yes, I just couldn't sit.

CB: With physical pressure in the body there's going to be movement. You need to relieve some of the discomfort.

Tamara: That makes sense, because I couldn't just sit. I kept in a movement thing.

CB: I'd say you were very successful, Mom.

Tamara: I think I was. I have a beautiful healthy boy. I like to think it's all perfect, with what was supposed to happen. It was an incredible thing.

CB: Do you feel that Calm Birth may have been helpful in dealing with pain and fear issues?

Tamara: Yes, it did really resonate with me in thinking about the fear of labor. I was afraid of that. But I do know that Calm Birth, just by listening to the tapes, you know, don't be afraid of the pain. Breathe with the contraction. Don't go against the contraction. That part of it made a lot of sense to me. Every time I would feel a contraction come on I was prepared for it. I was not totally welcoming the contraction, but I was leaning into it, and breathing into it, which I think helped me feel not totally out of control screaming. So that part was very helpful.

CB: [to David] What did you experience when you did the Calm Birth practices with Tamara? What do you remember?

David: I remember doing it with the intention to provide the right environment, or create the right intention, for the delivery of our baby. I'd say I experienced putting forth the right intentions with it.

Tamara: And that's how it was in the labor room too. Dave was really present, breathing with me. And it was great. For the whole labor thing I hope that the next time around I'll have a vaginal delivery and experience that feeling, but I'm okay if that doesn't happen too. It doesn't have to be a particular plan.

CB: You've done a courageous thing, I would say. Job well done, Mom.

Tamara: Thank you. I was proud of myself. And lying on the birthing table I was smiling. The doctor said, "Look, you're smiling." I felt radiant even then.... That's my experience. I was awake and talking. I felt connected to the doctors. It was a great experience.

CB: So as you reflect back on this, do you feel kind of like there was something about the spiritual aspect for you in the Calm Birth methods? I'm curious if you had anything that might stand out as a spiritual experience through some of the practices that you did prior to the delivery, or during or right after the delivery.

Tamara: Let me think. I know with the Calm Birth tapes when I would listen to them, it did take me into a space I loved, the tuning in to my womb and trying to visualize the light, and that little being growing inside of me. It was just incredible. The whole time I was thinking I was having a girl. So I wasn't totally aware [laughs] because it was a boy. And then of course we felt that when we conceived Mickey that it was a conscious conception. We were totally aware of what we were doing, of our intention. I did visualize a spirit kind of hovering above us, choosing us as its parents in this lifetime. Things like that would come to my mind. During the laboring process I remember at one point not resisting, but feeling fear; then I realized I was feeling that in my body and I said that I want to release that. I said I'm afraid to be a mother. I've never been a mother before. The responsibility was huge and I was aware of that during the contractions. I looked at the nurse, and I said something and I saw tears in her eyes. I said, Okay, I'm surrendering now. I'm ready to be a mom. Even when we're talking about it, it gives me chills because it was such a conscious place.

CB: How often did you do the practices at home on your own after taking the weekend intensive Calm Birth class and then attending the weekly classes?

Tamara: I knew I couldn't commit to doing it everyday, but it was always in my awareness. We did the practices together a few times a week. I think that the nurse who was first there with us at the hospital would have loved the Calm Birth practices. I think it's great for the nurses who are there because the doctors don't show up until the end.

CB: [to David] Could you envision the baby actually forming in Tamara's belly?

David: From the first moment, when we decided to conceive, we had a clear vision of creating a baby, at the exact moment we started trying. So that part was never difficult to envision.

CB: So you had that pre-birth experience, that spiritual experience when the conception happened?

David: Conscious conception experience, yes.

Tamara: I don't know if it was at exactly the same time; spiritually we were trying, envisioning the child at the same time. He's the ultimate joy, for sure. I never knew how much I could love.

CB: Did you or David have any meditation experience previous to the Calm Birth training?

Tamara: I had a very brief introduction to Buddhist meditation. Marina, one of the birth coaches, she did a Buddhist practice at her home, and I participated in that a little. I worked at that for a couple of months, and then I got pregnant. I did enjoy it.

CB: Do you feel like the Calm Birth practice and methods created any sort of direct bonding with the baby prior to birth, for you and with David?

Tamara: Yes, definitely yes. When I did the practice and I pictured the womb, and sending light to it, visualizing, it definitely was great, connecting me with what was going on inside my body, in a deeper level, feeding those blessings to it. That was really nice.

CB: How fortunate for the baby to have parents like you.

Tamara: Yes. To be present, that's what I wanted. I wanted to be as present as possible in his life. Because you often hear parents say it goes by like this [snaps her fingers]. You blink your eyes and then they're in high school. Gosh, I have to work part time, but when

I'm with him I want to know that I'm present and that he's being seen.

CB: How beautiful. That's incredible awareness you carry.

Tamara: Yes, thank you. There's a lot of our own self-discovery and personal work that's all part of it.

David: He's a very confident, comfortable baby.

Tamara: I think that's because of Calm Birth, and just being that conscious when he was being conceived and during the whole pregnancy, that's why he is so comfortable.... I did the deep belly breathing, which I visualized would help a baby in the womb. I did the *Womb Breathing* and sent the baby that energy. And I definitely was breathing that way as much as possible during the whole labor. I mean I had to.... I want to say that Calm Birth really enforced for me that I didn't have to do drugs. Which was great to have that. I would have friends who would say that you're crazy to not use painkilling drugs, just do it, like it's no big deal. Robert [Newman] was really good about giving us that information because I think if we have empowered mommas we have empowered babies. [laughs]

Elias John

JENNIFER AND MAX wanted to bring meditation into their lives. It was Jennifer's pregnancy and their desire for a natural childbirth that brought them to meditation in the Calm Birth program. They succeeded, meditating with their child in the womb throughout the pregnancy, labor, and delivery. Then they knew that meditation would be a good postnatal family path.

Parents: Jennifer and Max
Baby: Elias John
Birth date: February 25, 1999
Birth weight: 11 lbs 12 oz
Interviewers: Robert Newman and Whitney Wolf
Interview date: March 26, 2000

Postnatal Interview with Jennifer and Max

CB: You really applied the Calm Birth methods not only in the weekend training program but also on through the weekly follow-up classes. We know you were putting it in your systems. With respect to the reclining practice, we've had couples do that with the man visualizing the baby in himself. Did you do that, Max?

Max: Yes. It was pretty amazing. We used good thoughts and listened to the technique. Jennifer was doing it every night, but I was doing it probably every other night, right before bed usually.

CB: Did you have that experience of imagining the womb inside yourself?

Max: Yes, it was pretty awesome, amazing.... It allowed me to get a close bond with my child and it was nice that I could actually experience the pregnancy for all of us.

CB: How often did you practice the Calm Birth methods, Jennifer?

Jennifer: I did the practices every night meditating and focusing on my womb, focusing on the child. I developed a much stronger bond. It felt like I was feeding him energy and he was responding to it. So it felt like even though he was still in the womb I was caring for him. Our relationship was already being established. So, like when he came out it was like, I know you.

CB: You said you were sending him energy. You were one with him. Did you feel that energetically you were in meditation with the baby?

Jennifer: Yes.

Max: Oh, yes. We listened to the tape and that was our meditation practice. Instead of meditating on yourself, to focus your breath and all that, it was more focused on him, less on myself.

Jennifer: I didn't use the meditation techniques during the whole labor. I did use them more with the relaxing of the body. I did the practice of breathing directly into the area of the pain then, and it helped.

CB: Did you find that Calm Birth was a complement to what you were doing in your hospital class?

Jennifer: Definitely. I was going to try everything to have a natural childbirth. I wanted to really experience it.

CB: How often did you do the *Womb Breathing* practice?

Jennifer: I think about three times a week. It was early in the pregnancy that we started the Calm Birth program, in the fall. I was barely showing.... By the time of the birth the breathing practice was like an unconscious thing. It just became natural.

CB: So it had become like second nature?

Jennifer: Yes. And I think that definitely helped during the labor. I didn't even go to the hospital until I was eight centimeters dilated. I mean most people go in earlier than that.

CB: And your water broke at that point?

Jennifer: No, it never did.

Max: They thought of delivering him in it, but then at the last second the contractions started slowing down. They said it actually stopped in some cases. So they broke her water.

Jennifer: Yes, so I know the deep breathing helped throughout.... Yes, it was great. I couldn't have asked for anything better.

Max: There was all this smiling and then the baby came out and the doctor then came in just to catch the baby.

CB: Would you say that it was an easy birth?

Jennifer: Oh, no. I definitely went through some serious pain.

CB: There were some hard contractions?

Jennifer: Oh, yes. Then pushing was hard. It wasn't all just breathing. But then my contractions stopped in the pushing phase. That's when I think the primal stuff came out. [laughs]

CB: What made you think that it was time to go to the hospital?

Jennifer: That's when I realized, "Gosh, I'm really in pain here." My contractions were building. They were not consistently five minutes apart. It was like ten minutes then three minutes. Just not consistent.... It definitely was liberating. We look back and say, wow, we did that all by ourselves. It was just a process I took my body through.... I had friends who barely knew they were in labor. It wasn't that easy. But the only time I felt fear maybe was when I heard they wouldn't let you push for more than two hours and it was maybe getting to that time. The contractions weren't coming. So that was the only time I felt like, uh-oh, I hope the hospital doesn't want me to do a C-section. But I never really had the sense of what I'd call fear. When you give in to fear the problems start to arise.

CB: I think that's the most important thing, for a child to be born naturally without fear. It doesn't mean to be born without pain. It sounds like you worked with the pain well.

Jennifer: Yes. I could accept it.

CB: That affects the child importantly.

Jennifer: The doctor said he was very alert.

Max: The minute he was out of the womb he was wide-eyed, looking around. I didn't expect that. I think that's due to the calmness of the labor.

[Baby gleeful. Everyone laughs.]

CB: So you were instructed that meditation wasn't just for prebirth and birth. The more you continue to meditate, the more it will help the child in every way.

Jennifer: Max and I were thinking, you do all the prep work for the birth experience and then the hard part comes afterward. I think meditation's really good for him because he needs to calm down.

Emily Rose

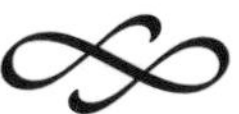

MARIE WAS A THIRTY-SEVEN-YEAR-OLD WOMAN with many medical problems when she became pregnant. She had prayed for a child in spite of the fact that she was told it would be impossible for her to conceive after she had been treated for ovarian cancer. She was told that if she did conceive it was unlikely that the child would be born, and if it was, she was warned, it might have serious health problems. When she did become pregnant she was encouraged to terminate the pregnancy. She refused. She was referred to the Calm Birth program both because Marie expressed interest in meditation and because her OB doctor thought that the Calm Birth program might help her in her high-risk pregnancy. Marie often did the Calm Birth practices for several hours a day. She and her husband Lee were exemplary in their commitment. They succeeded in having a natural childbirth. Marie became a teacher in the Calm Birth program and has helped bring the methods to many women the program otherwise may not have reached.

Parents: Marie and Lee
Baby: Emily Rose
Birth date: May 2, 1999
(approximately five weeks premature at thirty-three and a half weeks)
Birth weight: 4 lbs 4 oz
Interviewer: JoAnn Walker, RN
Interview date: March 23, 1999 [prenatal]

Prenatal Interview with Marie and Lee

CB: Would you please tell us your medical history before your pregnancy?

Marie: Okay. I have had several shunt revisions [a brain surgery that inserts a plastic tube into the brain and body cavities to drain the excess cranial fluid] because I was born with hydrocephalus, and I have intractable migraine syndrome, which means I don't know what it's like not to have a headache. Thanks to a lot of different techniques and technologies I can make my migraines much better. I have diabetes, chronic fatigue, TMJ, and a sleep disorder, narcolepsy, where I either sleep all the time or don't sleep at all, for weeks and weeks at a time. I have brain damage because of all the shunt revisions.

CB: When did the hydrocephalus start? [water on the brain; spinal fluid that does not drain on its own]

Marie: From birth. I had my first operation when I was twenty-seven days old. I'm not quite sure how many skull operations I've had, but I know it's over thirty.

CB: When were you diagnosed with diabetes?

Marie: 1984.

CB: And your hubby had been gone for a while? Almost three years?

Marie: Almost three.

CB: But you were still married, and he came home. There was supposedly no chance of you getting pregnant, right?

Marie: Virtually no chance, right.

CB: Yet it happened.

Marie: Yes. That's a real miracle.

CB: So here you are, you're thirty-seven years old and you've been told you can't get pregnant. You have multiple medical problems. You're on a variety of different medicines. And you're seven months pregnant?

Marie: Twenty-seven weeks. The doctor asked that I get tested right away, with ultrasound and stuff, because of all the medication I'm on, and all the different conditions. He wanted to know if abortion was an option. I told him it's just not an option with me.

CB: I think that's right. That child wants to come in.

Marie: Yes. I have only one fallopian tube and one ovary because of ovarian cancer. So it's even more of a miracle that I'm pregnant.

CB: Other than the surgeries for your shunts, you've had major abdominal surgery?

Marie: Yes.

CB: So you choose to work with an OB/GYN, and to continue your pregnancy.

Marie: Absolutely. It's a miracle. Because of all my medical conditions, and because of my history, I'm working very closely with my personal physician, and two different doctors in OB/GYN.

CB: Marie, you're considered a high-risk pregnancy. Your have a personal inclination to use alternative medicine, but with your situation you needed the help of both alternative and Western medicines. Because of your circumstances you're not going to be able to have a home birth, or have the birth in a smaller hospital. You're going to need more technology, which means going to a medical center. Marie, why will you probably need a medical center for the birth?

Marie: Because the hydrocephalus could go haywire.

CB: Do you have more fluid because you're pregnant?

Marie: Yes. They don't have a whole lot of knowledge yet. I was one of the first ones to ever get a shunt. What they do know is that pregnancies tend to clog shunts.

CB: So we've established your medical history before and after you became pregnant. The one intervention that we want to talk about here is Calm Birth. Marie, you and your husband, Lee, have attended the six-hour Calm Birth training and have attended the weekly hour support groups. I'd like you to tell us how often you do the Calm Birth practices? How are you using the Calm Birth childbirth methods?

Marie: Well, I use the Calm Birth audiocassette. I like both sides. I use the *Practice of Opening* to help me relax. Sometimes if the migraines aren't too bad, I practice both sides of the cassette. Sometimes I spend hours in the bathtub listening to the audioguide over and over again.

CB: So the Calm Birth cassette is helping you with relaxation. Does it help with your headaches?

Marie: Depending on the magnitude of the headache.

CB: In terms of doing the Calm Birth practices have you noticed any changes with the baby? Have you noticed her respond?

Marie: Oh, yes. She relaxes and settles down most of the time when I practice.

CB: You're teaching the Calm Birth method to some of your friends. How is that going, Marie?

Marie: We really like it because there is an audioguide. There is comfort in repetition. It's like listening to your favorite music. You can relax and it calms you sooner than just trying to calm yourself.

Lee: Marie's a very special woman. It's a miracle that she got pregnant with these different kinds of medications she's on. Medications and hormone shots will prevent a woman from getting pregnant. And in this particular case, God must want this baby to happen. Doctors tell her they're giving us less than 5 percent of a chance for us to have a child. But with the Calm Birth methods, it's helped us get closer together. And it helps us get closer to our child. That we can relate with. The baby will teach us a lot of things when she gets here. She's going to teach us how to be a parent. And we're going to teach her to have fun in life and to help other people when she gets older. The Calm Birth practices are helping us with our emotional needs. The practice helps us relax our physical bodies, and also helps us with our emotions, when we go through excitement. Tension, fear, and frustration rise up sometimes. The Calm Birth practices help us deal with it and realize that this life is a miracle that we're going through.

Postnatal Interview with Marie and Lee

Interviewer: Robert Newman
Interview date: May 7, 1999 [postnatal]

CB: Marie, were the Calm Birth methods an assistance to you in stopping your premature labor?

Marie: Yes. Yes. Primarily because I knew from practicing the Calm Birth audiotape and classes how to relax my body. That's very important.

CB: You were in labor but didn't realize it; can you tell us about this?

Marie: Yes. It didn't start being strong until about midnight. And then she was born at 6:25 in the morning, so it was a short and easy labor.

CB: Do you attribute that to Calm Birth?

Marie: Yes, primarily, because there were times where the pains would get bad enough so that I'd forget the *Womb Breathing*, and they had me pant like a puppy, and I found that all that did was make me feel like I was hyperventilating. So I remembered the Calm Birth teaching from the Calm Birth tape, and that helped me through labor immensely.... The practice had become like second nature.

CB: So you were in the hospital, in labor, and the practices, you say, were active in you spontaneously?

Marie: That is correct.

CB: What about the pushing part?

Marie: The more I was able to push, the less painful the contractions were, and I was able to push her out relatively quickly because I had fresh air, and I had normal breathing.

CB: What about the fears you had because of all the things that could go wrong?

Marie: I had been experiencing panic attacks the last couple of days, since I had been home from [the first premature labor visit to] the hospital, and I practiced the Calm Breathing then, and it helped a lot.

Nicholas

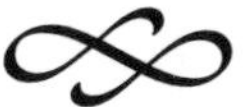

NORA'S FIRST CHILD was born in Argentina. She was anxious and isolated throughout that pregnancy, with no support and no childbirth education. Her husband wasn't allowed to be with her at the birth and she didn't know any of the birthing personnel at the hospital. She was given anesthesia and woke up the day after the child had been delivered by C-section. Several years later, with three months remaining in her second pregnancy, she met two of the Calm Birth teachers and began practicing the methods. Her second birth experience was very different from her first. As she tells us, she was able to have the birth she always wanted.

Parents: Nora and Javier
Baby: Nicolas
Birth date: May 26, 1999
Birth weight: 8 lbs 7 oz
Interviewers: Robert Newman and Colleen Graham
Interview date: May 2, 2000

Postnatal Interview with Nora

(Note: Colleen, one of the Calm Birth interviewers, was present at the birth as Nora's doula.)

CB: What inspired you to come to the Calm Birth program?

Nora: I was trying to have a better pregnancy than with my first child. I was trying to have a happier pregnancy. The first time, in Argentina, I was very nervous and insecure. The last month was sort of a nightmare. My mother wasn't with me, and I missed her. I felt anxious. There were many nights I couldn't sleep, not just sleepless, but sad, and thinking and thinking and thinking. Then I had a C-section. I'd never seen the doctor before. It was a very bad experience.

CB: I remember you saying you didn't have much of a birth experience. They gave you anesthetic and you woke up much later.

Nora: Yes. My husband wasn't allowed to be with me. I had no support at all.

CB: So this time you wanted to have much more support, and to be more empowered.

Nora: Yes. I had met with Colleen[11] and Sandra[12] on my birthday, and they said that I didn't have to do the same thing twice [C-section]. Then everything changed. I started relaxing and enjoying the pregnancy. I began to study at the university, to take more classes.

CB: The title, "Calm Birth," did that mean something to you?

Nora: Yes. But you have to be ready. Colleen said to sit down and relax, and I did. I wasn't a perfect student, like doing it every morning, but I did the practice.

CB: How often?

Nora: I had had a virus and was sick for two weeks, but when

---

11. Colleen Graham is a doula, educator, and Calm Birth teacher.

12. Sandra Bardsley, RN, is a midwife, educator, and Calm Birth advisor.

Colleen asked me to sit down and do the practice, from the first time I did it I felt better. It allowed me to not think, to put my mind at ease. To relax. I began to sleep better. I did it several times a week.

CB: There are two sides to the audiocassette. In the reclining practice, you go right into the womb with the child.

Nora: Yes.

CB: Did that help you in terms of actually making contact with the child?

Nora: Yes. Definitely. He is more outgoing than my first child. We had conversations when he was in the womb. He moved a lot. We felt very close. I remember the practices. The one where you lie down allowed me to relax and have good sleep at night, which I couldn't do with my first pregnancy. This time I was able to just focus on the baby and myself and the pregnancy.

CB: You mentioned about actually communicating with him in the womb, like speaking with him directly, in telepathic communication with the child. Women regularly have what are called paranormal experiences in childbirth.

Nora: Yes. I'll remember the joy of the communication. My first birth was so heavy. I'll never forget how joyful this second childbirth has been.

CB: Did the language on the Calm Birth cassette enable you to reach Nicholas and meditate with him?

Nora: Yes. Probably that's true. We're very connected. I think that the last two weeks, when the first contractions came, I put on the audiocassette and it really, really helped me. It relaxed me and helped me to focus on what was going on.

CB: That also helps the baby focus. You do the practice together. The resonance of that language as it's being spoken is for both the mother and the child. In making the cassette we imagined that the child would be listening with the mother, possibly with extraordinary awareness.

Nora: The labor was long. It ended up being a Cesarean, even though I wanted a natural birth. The breathing practices from the audiocassette were implemented during this time. I was in labor for two days. Finally I decided to have the C-section because the labor just wasn't working out. Because I felt relaxed, I felt okay with that, and he is a gifted child. That is communication, isn't it? He just loves communication. It doesn't matter what age they are, he just loves to be with people and he expresses his feelings perfectly well. His smile is something beautiful.

CB: So maybe the best thing for him was that communication that you gave him before birth. It was like a prayer being answered to bring him to his greater potential.

Nora: He is very responsive to music. And he's so beautiful. The doctor looked at him and said he was such a beautiful newborn. Exquisite and so nice and alert. His eyes were looking around. He wasn't cranky. Just an open baby.

CB: In the Calm Birth class at the hospital we talked with you about the method of breathing energies in the air to benefit the child in the womb. Were you able to do that during labor?

Nora: Yes. The labor was hard. I really tried the deep breathing. When I wasn't doing that I tried to focus, but I was busy with my first son the whole day. So I put the cassette on and communicated with the child, saying that he was really wanted. I told him he had a mother, a father, and a brother here who really want him, and love him. I did that every day. When I felt a contraction I was playing the cassette and saying, oh, we're so right for you, it's okay to come out.

CB: Are you saying that you were doing two things at once, breathing the precious energy from the air and sending love energy to him?

Nora: Yes. In the community hospital I did listen to the cassette once, with the birthing nurses, but other people came, visitors came. I did the deep breathing method during the labor. I couldn't imagine not doing it.

CB: After you were given the audiocassette at your birthday party, how long did it take you to realize that the methods were useful?

Nora: Two tries. Two times. The first time I thought it was okay, not so bad; but the second time I was sick, and so worried about the baby. When you're sick and pregnant the only thing you can take is Tylenol. But the audiocassette really helped me. It helped me to relax. That night I could just think of the baby and myself, and it was okay. To me, after the first pregnancy, feeling relaxed was a big thing. With the first birth I couldn't sleep for nights and nights.

CB: When you went to sleep at night, did the energy of the cassette stay with you?

Nora: Yes, absolutely.

CB: Because of that relaxation, at least as I noticed it in you, you were more confident about your pregnancy.

Nora: My pregnancy had a before and after. Before I met with Colleen and Sandra and got the cassette, I was insecure and afraid. I thought my first childbirth experience was repeating. But with the Calm Birth methods I realized I don't have to do that again. I relaxed and took the classes. I'd been so afraid that I didn't even mention to people that I was pregnant because the first experience had been so bad.

CB: So it sounds like your birthday party with Colleen and Sandra was the turning point.

Nora: Marie was there too so we were four women. They cooked dinner for me. It was like a special club that women have in being a mother. We were together in the joy of having a baby. I'd been sick and I went home and listened to the cassette and everything was different. Amazing. And my husband was very involved.

Colleen: I remember him saying, "Nora, remember your breathing. Breathe like you were guided on the audiocassette, *Womb Breathing*."

Nora: I tried it in different positions; the best one for me was on my knees. I was 100 percent focused. And my husband was right there, with his memory of the cassette. We did it all together. I couldn't imagine him not being there. He was the most committed, most dedicated husband I could imagine. And this is the product [holding up her baby, Nicholas].

CB: Nora, when do you think a pregnant woman should start practicing these methods?

Nora: I think the cassette is really good, and I think women need to use the cassette whenever they feel ready to have this commitment with themselves. As I learned during the famous conversation that day, being pregnant is a very special moment. It's okay to feel and to show everybody and to be proud of that. It is a very special moment. These nine months are a very special period in your lifetime. Because I was busy with my first child, the cassette helped me focus on the pregnancy, on the child inside me. So I thought, I want to be with the unborn child tonight, so I will put on the cassette and practice and be with him. I'm sure his open style is related to that experience. He had a different mother than my first child. With Nicholas, the eye contact and the communications are easier.

CB: He's calmer.

Nora: Exactly. They say the cassette helps you focus on your pregnancy, to stop everything, to say, I am pregnant. This is happening to me now and I will live this period of my life in the best way I can. The Calm Birth audioguide helps with that. I know pregnant women who act like nothing's happening.

Colleen: I noticed that when Nora would get kind of uptight, Javier, her husband, would say to her "Play the cassette and relax," and it would help. It gave him a tool.

Nora: Yes.

CB: So your husband's involvement and support during this childbirth was very important.

Nora: Yes. The experience with the first child was awful for both of us. There the doctors excluded him from the birth.

CB: The intention while creating the Calm Birth audioguide was that it's for both the mother and the father. Some couples do the Calm Birth practices with the couple lying side by side, going through their whole bodies together, with the man imagining the womb in himself. The woman's body and the man's body and the child's body became one.

Nora: Yes, the cassette really helps the father get closer to the child.

CB: How was Colleen there for you during your second pregnancy?

Nora: Colleen was my doula during the process. She was with me throughout the pregnancy and then for the three days before the birth. She was at the hospital with Javier and myself, exactly reminding me of my breathing.... I told Colleen that I saw a movie that when a baby was born they sang "Happy Birthday," and I loved that. And Colleen said we can do that. So we were in the recovery room, after the C-section, and everyone was happy, including the baby. And Colleen said, remember the birthday song! And we all sang happy birthday for him. The nurses were there. It was wonderful. The welcoming was very bonding.

Makai

Mysty and John were young honey farmers. It was their first pregnancy. They wanted a natural childbirth and connected with an OB doctor who was very supportive of the Calm Birth program. In preparing for the birth with the Calm Birth methods, Mysty and John had what they called fulfilling meditation experiences. They worked together closely as a birth team, using the methods throughout labor and delivery. They were very happy with the birth.

Parents: Mysty and John
Baby: Makai
Birth date: June 10, 1999
Birth weight: 8 lbs 3 oz
Interviewers: Robert Newman and Whitney Wolf
Interview date: January 22, 2000

Postnatal Interview with Mysty and John

Mysty: We were in our twenty-eighth week. We were looking for ways of giving birth where we could do it naturally. And I saw an announcement for a Calm Birth seminar. Up until that time I guess I was insecure about giving birth. I wondered whether I could do it without interventions. That wasn't possible with some doctors, but it was very possible with other doctors. So we were trying to figure out a way to do it without interventions, and we came across the Calm Birth announcement and we decided to take the seminar. It was very enlightening. It was two days long and we learned a lot. It was very insightful.

John: We learned and affirmed.

Mysty: Yes, learned and affirmed.

John: A lot of it was things we already believed. You gave back to us what we knew.

Mysty: We took the class and we learned a lot. I started using the audioguide, especially in the evening before I went to bed. And I actually had some really great meditation experiences, because I never used to meditate much and that was really cool.

CB: When you did the *Practice of Opening*, which is the reclining-relaxation part of our program, when you lie down and go through your whole body, it was our intention to help you bond with your unborn child. Childbirth research has shown that women spontaneously have natural spiritual experiences with the child, pre-birth experience and near-birth experience.

CB: Did you have anything like that?

Mysty: I did have some profound experiences, yes.

CB: What do you remember?

Mysty: I remember that I was meditating and I just felt real peaceful and kind of light. I should have written it down.

CB: What about the calm and the light? We emphasize the experience of light in the body. Is that what you meant by light?

Mysty: Yes, like light, luminous.

CB: John, did you sometimes do the cassette practice with Mysty?

John: Yes.

CB: You were supposed to visualize the womb within yourself. Did you do that?

John: Yes, we did that. We did that practice more than anything.

CB: You felt natural doing that?

John: Yes, absolutely. Definitely I felt the connection with her.

CB: Did you notice any difference in your experience after beginning the *Womb Breathing* practice?

Mysty: The only changes were that I felt more confident. Before I didn't know what to do. I was still frightened. With the methods it was almost like I had tools. I was armed with something I could use. Before that I had been at the mercy of whatever.

John: If it was only to make a person confident, that's a great thing to do for somebody. But I think it's more than that. Because if you really establish that connection with the unborn child, you focus your energy on that being, welcoming and nurturing.

CB: We know you had a quick labor. You had labor contractions and you called Dr. Olsen and you went straight to the hospital?

Mysty: Dr. Olsen said it probably wouldn't be that day. It would probably be the next day or the next day. It could be that day but it probably will be the next day. But we were primed for it because we knew.

John: Yes. I said I'm not starting any chore that I can't stop right away. I knew it was that close.

CB: What do you attribute that to, John, the awareness that you're speaking of?

John: Some of it probably stems from the meditation and having a good bond before he was out. Also the high level of communication between the two of us. It seemed like it was happening and it was.

CB: Did you say that the labor wasn't hard?

Mysty: It was relatively easy.

John: Not that easy.

Mysty: Yes, I catch myself saying it was easy, but I was in labor all day long. I was really excited.

John: The stuff that lasted all day long was mild. We went shopping.

Mysty: Dr. Olsen said go home. She was aware of where we live (twenty miles away from Ashland Community Hospital) and how long it would take to get back into the hospital. We went home. I called my mom. She said to walk around, but I was tired. We'd been home about half an hour. I decided to lie down and do some of the meditation.

John: She did some good visualization.

Mysty: Yes, I did some visualizations of my cervix opening. It was while I was doing that that my water broke and I went into intense labor. We went back to the hospital by the back roads.

CB: On the audiocassette it says, "Use this practice when labor comes. When labor comes, use this practice." Were there times when labor was happening that you remembered to use the Calm Birth methods?

Mysty: I didn't have to remember. I just did it, automatically. It's like I knew to do it. I'd catch myself doing the breathing already. And John was helping me as I did breaths.

John: It did get a little difficult because we wanted to incorporate *Womb Breathing.* At a certain point when they said they wanted her to push at it and do the panting, that was weird for me.

Mysty: Yes, that was hard for you, the nurses, yes.

CB: They weren't trained in our methods.

John: Everyone was looking at me like, how come you're not coaching the pant breathing, and I talked about this other kind of breathing we were trying to do.

Mysty: In the hard part of my labor I was in the Jacuzzi. I would start to pant when they told me to pant, and then I would slow down and just try to focus.

CB: They would say, "pant," fast-breathe, and you would want to slow down and focus?

Mysty: Yes.

John: If the nurses on duty had listened to the cassette it would have been different. . . . What I liked the most about your program is that before the baby is born you can communicate, bless and give it energy.

VII

New Childbirth Medicine

The new vision of the psyche . . . has far-reaching implications not only for each of us as individuals but for professionals in psychology and medicine.

—Stanislav Grof, *The Holotropic Mind*

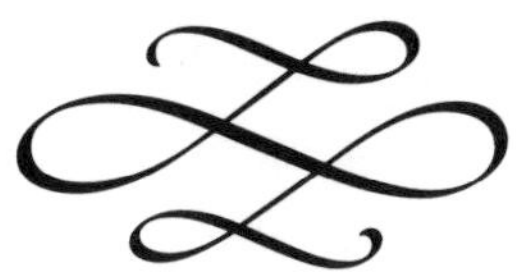

Meditation and the Nature of the Child

THOUGH VARIOUS FORMS OF ENERGY MEDICINE and mind/body medicine have been available as medical options for some time, childbirth science has been slow to accept such interventions. Though the methods Calm Birth is based on have been respected for a long time, their application in childbirth is new childbirth medicine.

Womb Breathing is both energy medicine and mind/body medicine applied to childbirth. It works by breathing energy into the energy body and by shifting from mind to awareness, a dual means of improving childbirth health. The application of progressive neuromuscular release *(Practice of Opening)* to childbirth may be the most important use of that proven mind/body method to date. The application of *Giving and Receiving* to childbirth is a new and important use of the revered method it is based on. All three methods have the potential to improve the quality of awareness and life force in the womb child and in his or her family.

In the practice of mindfulness-awareness meditation, such as *Womb Breathing,* people repeatedly shift their attention from mind to open awareness. In childbirth meditation pregnant women keep returning to the innate awareness they were endowed with, the innate awareness their womb child is endowed with. When a pregnant woman turns her attention to what is innate she touches upon our inherent unity in primal awareness, a deep basis for bonding. She knows that the profound awareness nature of her child and her own primal awareness nature are one.

Prenatal meditation helps the child maintain awareness as it is born and after it is born, an important basis of psychophysical health. A pregnant woman's prenatal meditation may inspire the child to be free of fear and have fearless confidence in awareness. Children are exposed to stressful experiences during pregnancy and delivery, as well as in infancy and childhood. The resource of its mother's prenatal meditation serves as a reference point for the child to return to its own calming connection with innate awareness.

When the mother practices postnatal meditation, the child is again reminded of its innate tendency to awareness, a key to health, survival, and meaningful engagement with life. Such children may have an inclination to meditation as a foundation of their personal development.

The relation of family and child through prenatal and postnatal meditation provides a foundation for a new and better society, a society of people willing to see many dimensions of life with awareness cultivated in meditation. The need for this quality of life is inseparable from the need for new childbirth methods that can make it inevitable.

Intention can be a vital energy resource for new childbirth medicine. When a pregnant woman practices prenatal meditation for herself and her child, by using intention as a force of nature she can meditate not only for herself, her child, and her family, but also for her society and all of life. That is the definite energetic potential of intention. In Buddhism it has been known and practiced as an invaluable resource for centuries. With the inevitable worldview given to everyone today by omnipresent media communications, through the unlimited potential of intention a woman meditating to benefit herself and her child can benefit the world. Such intention will encourage the birth of indigo children and crystal children, children born with fully developed awareness and wisdom, savants, wise ones, born for the sake of the planet. The intention to benefit all life is inherent in such children coming in.

Benefits of Prenatal Audioguidance

ALL THE RESEARCH CITED BELOW concerning hearing in the womb is from the work of David Chamberlain (1998):

> Signs of ear development can be seen in your prenate only a week after conception. By the halfway mark of pregnancy, elaborate labyrinths, chambers, and passageways with impressive nerve and brain connections are in place. . . . Since other parts of the baby's brain and nervous system are only partially insulated at birth, it seems that hearing has a very high priority (p. 22).

The womb is a sound chamber in which there is constant infant hearing response, to the sounds of the woman's body, and to external sound, which it perceives directly. The infant is particularly sensitive to the sound of its mother's voice. Her words, her songs, her sighs, her laughter radiate throughout her body. Sound is transmitted remarkably well through the liquids of her body, through her womb. The sound is louder and clearer than we might imagine. The infant may also hear through bone conduction.

For the pregnant woman practicing the meditative energy of the audioguide, prenatal audioguidance may help neutralize negative conditioning before birth. The infant hears physically and in sympathetic resonance with the woman. Verbal communication before birth, including words the mother is listening to carefully, can inspire a higher level of communication and awareness in the womb child. This may result in more advanced language abilities in the child.

> Appropriate audio therapy in the perinatal period can positively influence the state of consciousness and protect from an inappropriate stress response. This gives us an opportunity to impart our love as well as our wisdom. The implications are that these modalities will lead to physical and emotional benefits to the mother and newborn as well as medical cost savings (Schwartz, 1997, p. 27).

The womb child with the experience of prenatal audioguidance will be energetically in sympathetic resonance with its mother's attention to that voice and it will hear that voice directly. That child will be born familiar with a voice encouraging intelligence.

Advances in audio technology make it possible to hear the recorded human voice more clearly than it has ever been heard. In the third edition of the Calm Birth prenatal methods, CB3 (2005), attention is engaged by the voice of the transmission with more potential impact than has been possible in earlier offerings of audio-guidance. In the advanced edition of the Calm Birth methods, the voice of transmission is heard vividly by woman and womb child, a voice encouraging a breakthrough in childbirth health.

Paranormal Childbirth Experience

MANY BOOKS AND PAPERS have been published about normal people having paranormal experiences, experiences of great ability and realization. Many of the reported paranormal experiences occur in near-death situations, where people experience being all-knowing, all-seeing, having marvelous powers, being full of unforgettable transformation.

Books have also been written researching paranormal childbirth experience. Women have precognition, are sometimes clairvoyant, and have remarkable states of illumination in childbirth. With new, noninvasive childbirth methods, there is a dual increase in the potential for extraordinary experience, for the woman and for the child. The methods help women avoid unnecessarily medicated birth, which limits the potential of awareness and realization, and they offer woman and child ways to more fully access the developmental experience potential of childbirth.

Regarding childbirth offering paranormal birth potential, Danah Zohar, celebrated MIT and Harvard professor of physics and philosophy, now at Oxford, writes:

> During the pregnancy of my first child, and for some months after her birth, I experienced what for me was a strange new way of being. In many ways I lost the sense of myself as an individual, while at the same time gaining a sense of myself

> as part of some larger and ongoing process.... At first the boundaries of my body extended inward to embrace and become one with the new life growing inside me. I felt complete and self-contained, a macrocosm within which *all* life was enfolded.... During those months, "I" seemed a very vague thing, something on which I could not focus or get a grip, and yet I experienced myself as extending in all directions, backwards into "before time" and forwards into "all time," inwards toward all possibility and outwards towards all existence ... (Zohar, 1990, pp. 141–147).

Elizabeth Hallett, researcher in paranormal birth experiences, published the account of a woman who reports, "I had gone to sleep feeling very peaceful and comfortable with my pregnancy; almost in a meditation state. Upon waking, the clearest dream-vision was overpowering in my memory. I was seeing through my son's bright blue eyes—his hands drifting through the pale fluid. Then I was seeing his face. Large blue eyes; almost translucent skin, ears, nose, eyelids ..." (Hallett, 1995, p. 54). This kind of experience is explicitly encouraged by *Practice of Opening.*

Practice of Opening is designed to inspire paranormal childbirth experience. It encourages extraordinary seeing and knowing. It can enable people to see on a cellular level and know life force directly, and it can facilitate direct communication with the womb child. *Womb Breathing* encourages recognition and use of energy systems designed for function and capability beyond ordinary ranges of activity. *Giving and Receiving* helps women recognize and use their ability to transform their sense of body and capability, in childbirth and beyond.

Eventually near-birth experiences may be considered as important a part of the legend of human life as near-death experiences.

Postnatal Healing and Care

WE KNOW THAT POSTPARTUM CHALLENGES may include depression as well as anxiety. The causes may be unnatural birth interventions such as anesthesia, drugs and surgery, and other factors, such as heightened anxiety in the world. The more adverse the impact of medical interventions in childbirth the greater the need for postnatal meditation. New postpartum methods are needed as much as prenatal methods. They are deeply needed to heal depression and the various results of birth shock and trauma caused by prevailing obstetrical practices. Postnatal meditation strengthens the immune system to heal the side effects of birth drugs and anesthesia and helps heal the wounds of birth-related surgery. It may also release psychological harm caused by obstetrical forces. Methods such as *Vase Breathing,* which is *Womb Breathing* when there is no child in the womb, are particularly effective as both energy medicine and mind/body medicine applied to postnatal care.

Meditation is an antidote to depression. It produces feel-good endorphins, which women generate through their will to do the practice, giving themselves self-regulated release from negative mental and emotional states. As an antidote to depression, meditation offers a method to intentionally shift from obstructive emotions and thoughts into open awareness, saving energy and building new energy. This energy may bring a sense of wellness and confidence. Sitting meditation, in general, tends to bring a revolution in attitude that can be vital in relieving depression. Sitting upright balanced in a stable, calm posture counteracts the body language of depression and touches upon inherent psychological freedom. Also, postnatal reclining meditation enables women to restore reserves that may have been depleted from childbirth.

Meditation cultivates important hormonal benefits that help

women counteract possible adverse health impacts of medical interventions used in the delivery process. Those same hormonal benefits of meditation are given to the child through breast-feeding, helping the child reduce and eliminate possible adverse impacts of medical interventions.

Not only does the meditating woman give immune-system-enhancing hormonal benefits to her child through lactation and breast-feeding, women who meditate after giving birth influence the infant to be calm. The child "picks up" the meditative energy of the mother. With maternal and/or paternal meditation support, children will tend to be healthier physically and psychologically, and tend to have an interest in meditation.

The Calm Birth program offers three methods for postnatal care. (Visit the Calm Birth web site for more detail: www.CalmBirth.org.) These methods are both for women who have practiced the prenatal Calm Birth methods and for women who may come to the Calm Birth postnatal methods having been through a turning point in their lives, finding that it is time to train in empowering methods. The women who use these methods want to provide a healthy energy field for themselves and for their children.

Calm Birth also offers a movement program for postnatal empowerment. It includes tantric dance and sacred movements disclosed by Carlos Castaneda, the *Magical Passes.* A major series of those movements, *The Series for the Womb,* was designed centuries ago to enable women to realize their unique abilities to see energy and to use their uterus and ovaries as "the epicenter of evolution" (Castaneda, 1998, p. 72).

The above postnatal methods can be considered energy medicine, mind/body medicine, and energy body movement for physical, psychological, and spiritual postnatal health.

Meditation Methods and Research

CHARACTERISTICS OF THE VARIOUS KINDS of meditation available from different meditation traditions prevalent in the West vary substantially, but the published results of more than fifteen thousand studies and books clearly indicate important benefits. The research on DHEA elevation was determined on the basis of Transcendental Meditation (TM), a mantra-based technique. The research on melatonin elevation was determined on the basis of Buddhist mindfulness-insight meditation, a psychological method. Further research would probably show that each method produces elevated levels of both hormones.

The Calm Birth method of the *Practice of Opening* will tend to yield results similar to those observed in Jacobson's work (1938) and in Kabat-Zinn's program (1990); but the *Practice of Opening* audioguidance language was developed to produce new benefits.

Similarly, the practice of *Womb Breathing* exhibits benefits similar to those observed in Buddhist *Vipashyana* (mindfulness) practice; yet *Womb Breathing* has dimensions that give the practice additional potential. Though based on the traditional practice of *Vase Breathing*, *Womb Breathing* is a new method inspired by meditation science and by the needs of childbirth medicine. Benefits of *Womb Breathing* need to be observed through ongoing clinical application. Research protocols are being prepared.

The method of *Giving and Receiving* is based on the Buddhist practice of *Ton Len*, proven effective for centuries and now used widely in medical application. Yet *Ton Len* still has not been significantly researched in the West. With respect to its new application in the Calm Birth program, and with respect to all three complementary Calm Birth methods, one intention of this writing is to draw interest and support for research in childbirth meditation in general.

But before medical science can advance enough to evaluate the benefits of methodologies such as Calm Birth, it must appreciate its foundations in greater science, science as the search for truth, and it must see that such "deep science" (Wilber, 1999) is in fundamental unity with the principals of meditation science.

> Where the exemplar in the physical sciences might be a telescope, and in the mental sciences might be linguistic interpretation, in the spiritual sciences the exemplar, the injunction, the paradigm, the practice is: meditation or contemplation. It too has its injunctions, its illuminations, and its confirmations, all of which are repeatable—verifiable or falsifiable—and all of which therefore constitute a perfectly valid mode of knowledge acquisition (p. 170).

Contemporary EEG studies of meditative states, continues Wilber, show that meditation

> ... produces dramatic and repeatable changes in the entire organism, and most significantly in the electrical patterns of the brain itself, presumably the seat of consciousness (p. 198).

> To check or refute the claims of meditation science, investigators will have to use deep science: namely, take up the injunction or paradigm of meditation; gather the data, the direct experience, the apprehensions that are disclosed by the injunction; compare and contrast the resultant data with that of others who have completed the first two strands. (Those who refuse this injunction are simply not allowed to vote on the truth of the proposition, just as the churchmen who refused to look through Galileo's telescope were not competent to form an opinion about the existence of the moons of Jupiter.) (p. 199).

VIII

Toward a New Era of Childbirth Education

The human being, in essence, is in the process of discovering self-responsibility and personal empowerment. These two newly emerging characteristics contain the necessary seeds for creating an entirely new global society.

—Norman Shealy and Caroline Myss, *The Creation of Health*

Both spontaneously and through transformational practice, a new evolutionary domain is rising in the human species.

—George Leonard and Michael Murphy, *The Life We Are Given*

Seen with new eyes, our lives can be transformed from accidents into adventures. We can transcend the old conditioning.... We have new ways to be born.

—Marilyn Ferguson, *The Aquarian Conspiracy*

Toward a New Era of Childbirth Education

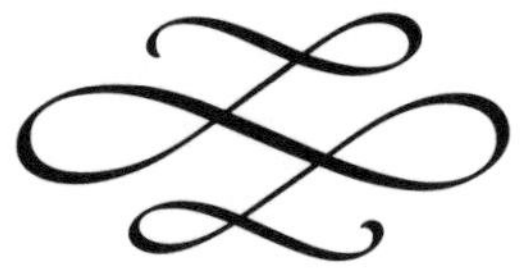

Introduction

In childbirth medicine today, through the widespread use of anesthesia and pain-blocking chemicals, awareness is suppressed in the large majority of the childbirths in the industrialized countries. Although the medical establishment may believe that the reduction or elimination of awareness of labor pain is a compassionate intervention, and though chemically induced calm may allow other interventions that make the process of childbirth convenient for doctors and lucrative for hospitals, the routine suppression of awareness in childbirth may be diminishing the evolutionary quality of the human species. In the large majority of births women do not function in the way they were made to naturally function, and they are unaware as that happens.

This is a pivotal concern for a needed revolution in childbirth education. Quality of awareness may be the most essential concern in childbirth. Suppression of awareness in childbirth interferes with maternal and infant health. The recognition, cultivation, and protection of dual prenatal awareness may be the most essential challenge to childbirth science today. The shift in the medical paradigm lets us see the problem deeply and lets us see the possibility for radical change in childbirth methodology and education.

Establishing the Value of Awareness in Childbirth

Understanding that the awareness of the woman and the child is most often suppressed by prevalent labor interventions that have biological and psychological risks, we need to establish a new priority of respect for the awareness of the pregnant woman and of the child in the womb. Natural childbirth is founded on prenatal awareness. Natural childbirth programs empower women to remain aware, trust their innate capability, and make choices that will protect their right to give birth naturally. This supports access to important developmental experiences in the process of childbirth, sometimes including paranormal experience, while avoiding interventions that take away that potential.

The childbirth experience is an opportunity for parents and prenates to strengthen and develop psychologically. Natural childbirth training is not just about how to tolerate labor pain. It enables women to appreciate the intelligence of labor contractions and to come into expanded awareness in the process of a joyous birth (Odent, 1994). Various exercises, particularly breathing exercises, are offered in natural childbirth classes to preserve the integrity of awareness and natural capability, although programs presented by Dick-Read (1944), Lamaze (1958), and Bradley (1965) have not emphasized the full potential of awareness and realization in childbirth.

Today, with the increasing availability of meditation methods in the West, more and more women come to pregnancy with a developed sense of the nature of awareness from meditation experience. Such women would choose childbirth education in which meditation training was an important option, if it was available. With meditation practices based on a more profound knowledge of breathing and awareness, we could be on the threshold of a new era of natural childbirth. Advanced childbirth education incorporating meditation science supported by more sensitive medical protocols could offer women a new level of childbirth experience and health and protect the evolutionary quality of the species as well.

Use of the word *science* in conjunction with the word *meditation* reflects the fact that both Buddhist and Hindu meditation traditions are based on centuries of experience with highly refined methods and knowledge of their psychological and physiological consequences. Extensive literature exists, much of it in excellent translation now and accessible internationally, illuminating the methods of this science. That literature is revered and is the basis of great teaching traditions. Buddhism, particularly, has always called itself a science of human development rather than a religion. In its meditation science, psychological phenomena are observed from a basis of invaluable experience and sophisticated methodology. As Wilber has said (see Chapter VII), meditation science has adhered to the deepest principals of science. In comparison, some of the most vaunted 20th century sciences, for lack of vision, have plunged this planet into the gravest of dangers, while meditation science has proven beneficial through the ages, doing no harm but much good.

Professional medicine and childbirth education have the opportunity to work with meditation science and psychological sciences in general to make decisive improvements in childbirth values.

The Medical Paradigm and Awareness

Before going further, we must consider the changes taking place in the medical establishment that will make it possible to create a new quality of childbirth education and birth.

A reductionist form of medicine (also called material, mechanical, or physical medicine) has dominated medical science for at least one hundred years (Dossey, 1993). This form of medicine holds tenaciously to the idea that human consciousness is a product of the brain.

From this limited perspective the brain of a human fetus is considered incomplete, the brain of a newborn still immature, and intelligence or awareness is unexpected until months or years after birth. This justifies aggressive medical interventions during labor and delivery, during postpartum routines in hospital care, as well as during surgery at all phases including intra-uterine surgery, surgical delivery, and major surgery postpartum. In prevalent birth medicine, there is the presumption that no infant learning or memory will occur in either the prenatal or perinatal period. This means that doctors and nurses, however compassionate they may be as individuals, offer care constrained by accepted medical beliefs and values they were taught in school.

Fortunately, in the last few decades, medical science has been expanding its understanding of the infant senses, including the reality of infant pain perception, and has begun to consider that there might be a level of development that includes emotion and thought associated with the infant brain. Now, with important developments in the medical paradigm in the past three decades, mind/body medicine is included in medical and nursing education, a trend affected by a strong surge of public opinion in its favor. Such medicine has a fundamental interest in infant awareness, which may be present as early as conception, and a strong interest in the use of meditation in childbirth to respect and advance prenatal intelligence.

Currently, meditation is being extensively researched and broadly confirmed as a "new" science, although it has a very long history in which it has been repeatedly tested. This ancient method and its wisdom offer tools that could revolutionize natural childbirth. Meanwhile, childbirth education as presented under medical auspices still limits the tools it offers pregnant women, and encourages epidural anesthesia, chemical pain blocks, and C-sections as right and reasonable childbirth choices. Those interventions have risks, evidenced by the malpractice lawsuits that have shaken the business of obstetrics. It is imperative to incorporate new guidelines and higher values, along with women's rights to natural childbirth options, in appropriate childbirth education. What is missing in the current curriculum is the value and appreciation of awareness, and the low-risk methods that bring natural, self-induced calm to the drama of childbirth.

Awareness and Life Itself

ADULTS AND CHILDREN can directly experience the timeless and open quality of awareness at any moment. Children can readily learn meditation. They have a knack for experiencing open awareness, probably because it's inherent. Although we don't have the technology to reveal mental states in womb children, their awareness may be innate. Therefore, it would be prudent to give them the benefit of the doubt and respect their consciousness.

> Consciousness, in order to manifest, depends on billions of processes in the organic body that humans have not even begun to understand. Each and everything in the cosmos is conscious in its own way. Atoms, molecules, cells, organisms, all have a sentience of sorts, and this consciousness becomes greater and greater the higher in evolution you go (Wilber, 2002, p. 444).

In sensing that awareness may be innate in the moment of human conception, innate in the embryo, we can sense the immanence of intelligent forces of great magnitude required to produce the embryo of an embodiment designed to carry a potentially great awareness.

Self-awareness is probably a very early experience of the fetus. In fact, evidence of awareness and intelligence is being noted at earlier and earlier stages of development (Verny, 1981, 2002; Chamberlain, 1998, 1999). David Chamberlain's statement is pivotal:

> Prenatal/perinatal memories are transpersonal in transcending all the expected boundaries of consciousness during intra-uterine time and birth, especially memory, learning, sensation, emotion, perception, thought, dreaming, out-of-body experience, near-death experience, clairvoyance, and telepathy. None of these phenomena of consciousness were

> anticipated in the materialistic paradigm of 20th Century developmental psychology. In fact they were rejected ... (Chamberlain, 1999, pp. 86–87).

It is time to consider how intelligence may manifest itself from conception onward. This would be consistent with the combined insights of quantum physics, Buddhist meditation science, and transpersonal psychology.

It is not the intent of this writing to offer documentation from quantum physics pertaining to the creation of the universe, matter, and human conception, but to emphasize insights of revered scientists about the nature of these things. For instance, though Einstein (1954) was never satisfied that his Theory of Relativity was proven, his personal insights into the nature of the universe are of great value to us. This writing will call attention to some insights of renowned scientists that clarify our vision of conception. We look to teachings such as the Buddhist science of rebirth and the new field of scientific research corroborating past-life experiences, but we wish to focus on the essential quality of awareness that may be present at the moment of conception and in intra-uterine life. It may prove to be true that awareness is integral to or identical with the life force, and may be the foundation of life itself, the foundation of spirit or soul. As we shall see, renowned scientists say that awareness precedes matter and may create matter. The energy of awareness may precede the energy of spirit or soul.

Knowledge and the Moment of Conception

MEDICAL SCIENCE has been characteristically devoted to observable phenomena and physical evidence. However, with the advent of quantum physics, "observation" has been shown to be more subjective than objective, and can influence the phenomena observed. Thus, observation can be exposed as self-serving projection—a sobering fact in the quest for true knowledge. At the least, this is pushing science to a new appreciation of psychic and spiritual phenomena and the various dimensions of consciousness suggested by psychologist William James (1902/1961).

The fact that no technology has been created to observe the nature of awareness at conception is not important. What is important is that science, in its quest for true knowledge, has become more intuitive and telepathic, making use of various dimensions of consciousness. Some scientists look increasingly to ancient wisdom and its profound vision of reality.

Since a large majority of people, including most great spiritual teachers and many renowned scientists, believe in reincarnation, traditional and current knowledge of that important subject can help many of us understand the nature of awareness that is incarnating at conception.

Indeed, reincarnation may be the most important fact of life, and one that can be known directly through inherent human capability. Transpersonal conscious recall of the moment of conception and other early embryonic experiences have in fact been obtained in meditation, in spontaneous recall by young children, in the process of regression therapies, in hypnotherapy, in body psychotherapies, in LSD-assisted psychotherapy, and in various other altered-state experiences.

The Nature of Awareness

In contemporary science it is common to use the word *mind* as equivalent to *consciousness* or *awareness*. From the point of view of meditation science we can distinguish between mind and awareness. Awareness is innate cognitive capability, including intuition. It is an act of knowing. Awareness is probably an essential characteristic of the universal field and as such is often referred to as universal mind. In that context, energy has been seen to be essentially intelligent (Chopra, 1989). Human awareness is first and foremost awareness of itself. It is capable of being cognizant of itself and of external phenomena at the same time.

Mind is more difficult to define. It constantly changes. It's discontinuous. It thinks and speaks about itself frequently. It has genetically based qualities and qualities developed after infancy through language and other cultural experiences. Some energies of mind may be caused by reincarnation. In the following statements by renowned scientists, the word *mind* is used for what in childbirth we're calling awareness. Please be patient with that.

Life sciences, such as biology and medicine, are not used to dealing with nonmaterial entities like mind, but physics is. In the advance of science in the 20th century the world enthusiastically received the work of great physicists, including Einstein, Schrodinger, Margenau, and Bohm, who were able to explain mind as a field affecting matter but not caused by it. Dossey comments:

> What has happened is that biologists, who once postulated a privileged role for the human mind in nature's hierarchy, have been moving relentlessly toward the hard-core materialism that characterized nineteenth century physics. At the same time, physicists, faced with compelling experimental evidence, have been moving away from strictly mechanical models of the universe to a view that sees the mind as playing an integral role in all physical events (Dossey, 1989, p. 162).

In contrast to a biologist or medical scientist who is not interested in the new medical paradigm, or who is opposed to it, still insisting that mind is a product of brain function, Dr. Margenau observes,

> The nonmaterial mind [with the properties of a field] may be completely free and independent from the physical brain, yet fully capable of influencing it, without having to furnish any of the energy required in the transaction between the two. In very complicated physical systems such as the brain, the neurons and sense organs, whose constituents are small enough

> to be governed by probabilistic quantum laws, the physical organ is always poised for a multitude of possible changes, each with a definite probability; if one change takes place that requires energy ... the intricate organism furnishes it automatically. Hence, even if the mind has anything to do with the change, that is, if there is a mind-body interaction, the mind would not be called on to furnish energy (Margenau, 1987, p. 165).

But where does the mind come from if not from the brain? And if it comes from the universal field, what is individual mind as it may appear at conception and influence the development of the zygote? To the Nobel Prize laureate physicist Erwin Schrodinger (1969), mind is universal and immortal. Any individual mind *is* the universal mind. Mind is one mind, transpersonal, timeless, and nonlocal.

Nobel Prize laureates Einstein, Godel, and Bohm all agree that "Deep down the consciousness of all mankind is one; and if we don't see this it's because we're blinding ourselves to it" (Dossey, 1989, p. 175). The agreement of these eminent scientists is that not only is there a unification of awareness in its universal nature, but it is also, in its essential nonlocality, immortal. Being free of time and space are qualities that self-awareness perennially experiences in itself. Dossey states: "Ultimately all the moments are really one ... therefore now is eternity ... everything, including me, is dying every moment into eternity and being born again" (p. 176).

What they are not distinguishing, but what meditation science distinguishes, is that innate mind is both mind and awareness. Awareness has essential freedom from time and space that is a healthful basis for cognitive function in responding to the intense demands of human time and space, the life we are born into. Mind is chaotic, ego-centered thought, intensely concerned with time. Awareness, with its intuitive and open quality, provides a basis for the experience of timeless freedom.

Physics is respected by medical and psychological science for using rigorous, mathematical criteria. But history is changing faster than it ever has, and in part because of quantum physics, science is becoming more spiritual. In observing the nature of awareness, meditation science may be superior to physical science in distinguishing between mind and awareness and experiencing directly. Mind is derived from awareness, which is more fundamental. Meditation is able to know how inherent awareness is obscured by mind and it may offer freedom from reincarnated psychological obstructions as well as freedom from psychological obstruction developed in the present lifetime.

In brief, based on centuries of observation with the full resources of perennial wisdom essential to the evolutionary quality of the species, meditation science affirmed, previous to quantum physics, that awareness is innate, universal, timeless, primordial, immortal, and unlimited in cognitive potential. Meditation science was established in times less disturbed psychically, with more psychological stability, therefore with clearer vision. Its knowledge is as pertinent today as ever. Meditation science can help us recognize the dimensions of intelligence present at conception. Tarthang writes:

> The knowledge of how to control the mind to shape the process of rebirth has been passed on by the great lineage holders of the past. There are works that describe in detail practices for taking rebirth knowingly and how to perfect and refine this capacity of mind through meditation much as a chemist might use chemical reactions possible only under rarified conditions to create a new molecule (Tarthang, 2002, p. 92).

The increasing presence in the West of meditation science is an important resource for an expanded vision of childbirth science. Furthermore, the fact that 72 percent of Americans polled believe in reincarnation (Rosen, 1997) indicates that public interest in the nature of what incarnates warrants a change in childbirth education in which the recognition of awareness present as early as conception is the basis of new childbirth methods and values.

What Incarnates?

THE HUMAN EGG AND SPERM unite to form the zygote, millions and millions of living molecules, all of them vitalized by powerful atoms. Inside the atomic function of the zygote is open space and electric force. Inside that atomic space is universal quantum field, the life potential, completely aware.

The human zygote may receive aware incarnation as it is formed. For an instant awareness may be incarnated in a single cell, in its live quantum field. And then the cell starts to multiply dynamically forming embodiment. The incarnation may occur at conception or afterward. In the sacred knowledge of Tibetan Buddhist wisdom, at the moment of conception the universal and individual basis of aware life enter the zygote. In other ancient wisdom traditions, the conscious soul or spirit is seen to enter the embryo at a later stage of its development, or to enter the child with her or his first breath. What is important is that life may continue through death into life again, and that the timeless and deathless quality of awareness can be directly experienced.

At this point in the history of our species we can acknowledge a number of well-known facts about the status of reincarnation as we consider the question, "What incarnates?" According to Stanislav Grof (1993), major traditions, such as Buddhism and Hinduism, some important sects of Judaism and Christianity, schools, and various other orders, have been firm believers in reincarnation, in the continuity of life after death, and in rebirth. Such conviction is based on profound knowledge that is considered sacred. In the West, a large majority of people accept reincarnation, despite Roman Catholic doctrine that declares it a heresy. Other branches of Christianity are free to believe or disbelieve, but an increasing number embrace reincarnation.

The current widespread belief in reincarnation means that most pregnant women and their partners would be interested in knowing more about what incarnates. Childbirth professionals should therefore be more educated on this subject and be more ready to appreciate how it may relate to the entire process of conception, pregnancy, and birth. Since most sacred knowledge says that life reincarnates, sensitivity to the dimensions of what incarnates can be the basis of increased respect for the prenatal process, respect that may be cultivated through new educational norms.

Often children are remarkably unlike their parents. Many people have nonordinary experiences in which they engage one or more past lives, which are sometimes confirmed. People sense that something does incarnate that has both a spiritual and a biographical continuity, so that the genetic basis alone is an insufficient explanation of what happens at conception and afterward. It is important to respect that various people in nonordinary states of consciousness, inherent super-consciousness, have been able to know directly what incarnates.

> Research in transpersonal psychology continues to provide ample evidence that this area of study is a veritable treasure trove of insights into the nature of the human psyche. So convincing is the evidence in favor of past life influences that one can only conclude that those who refuse to consider this to be an area worthy of serious study must either be uninformed or excessively narrow-minded (Grof, 1993, pp. 126–127).

Generally it is assumed that people reincarnate for reasons related to their own spiritual growth or lessons to be learned. Some believe that a form of "contract" exists behind the choice of family members based on past relationships. Others who incarnate may be coming to relieve suffering in the world. In the Buddhist tradition this is known as a *"bodhisattva,"* one who has taken a vow to reincarnate in compassionate service to all life.

Some parents, ancient and modern, have prepared spiritually

to become pregnant and welcome a child soul into their life. Often they are able to directly perceive the moment of conception. Today there is a growing literature of parent reports of how their babies contacted them in meditations, visions, dreams, or other altered state experiences to tell them of their wish to join the family (Hallett, 1995). This is a somewhat common incidence of paranormal childbirth cognition that experiences awareness as integral to the soul or spirit incarnating. In this well-documented maternal experience, supported by significant anecdotal evidence, spirit or soul, life force, and awareness are inseparable.

At this time, when women and children are most often anesthetized and/or drugged in labor and delivery, appropriate childbirth education can be based on respect for the potential presence of awareness from the moment of conception onward, and the need to give women the option of childbirth with awareness. It's a matter of health and evolution.

The Need for Natural Childbirth Options

POSSIBLE PROBLEMS CAUSED by the suppression of awareness in childbirth may be viewed in different ways. First, if awareness is reduced or eliminated to avoid labor pain, the fear of pain may be strengthened, and a tendency to use pain-blocking agents may be imparted to the child being born. This may later contribute to addiction and extend the fear of pain. A consequence to the birthing woman is loss of her opportunity to prove her innate capacity for pain management in labor, and loss of opportunity to make her spirit more vital.

Today, women sometimes confess to feeling humiliated or cheated out of a normal birth experience after being routinely subjected to a series of medical interventions, depriving them of personal power and meaning. In those cases the interventions are depressing and are bad for the woman's psychological and physiological health and probably adversely impact her child. Due to cultural norms and inclinations, many women, particularly out of fear of pain, choose medicated birth without hesitation.

Though advances in birth medicine can be very helpful in some cases, the World Health Organization continues to warn that the innovations used are often unproven as to their safety, hence the many malpractice lawsuits. Birth medication often comes into the child in high dosages, administered according to the woman's body weight, as if the hospital administration didn't know how to be responsible to the child. Some of the drugs that have been used are known to be toxic. Since the infant's liver is not yet fully developed, she or he has been overwhelmed both with high dosages and the kinds of chemicals that have been used (Davis-Floyd, 2003, p. 99). "ANY medication reaching the baby may be too much" (p. 175). Medicated birth has risks, and though informed consent is essential, women are rarely fully informed about the risks.

For illuminating the variety of traumas caused by unaware professionals and parents in the prevalent way of birth, we can thank contributors to the *Journal of Prenatal and Perinatal Psychology and Health,* Volumes 1–19, from 1986 to the present. Practitioners in this new field are working to create new forms of therapy to resolve primal wounds, beginning as early as conception. For a broad and knowledgeable assessment of birth around the world we can thank Dr. Marsden Wagner. His important work for the World Health Organization has helped expose the tragic risks that come with unnatural childbirth.

Drugs tend to remove the mother's attention that contraction pain would be focusing exactly on the child in its descent. This results in a psychic abandonment of the child caught in the muscular contractions of its mother's body. In contrast, the light of uninterrupted caring attention focused by the mother on her child during labor and delivery may be sustained most gracefully by the use of sacred breathing techniques that allow the child uninterrupted mindful connection with the mother during the birth process.

The present availability of such techniques in childbirth helps to enrich and extend natural childbirth options. Appropriate childbirth education could be based on recognition and support of innate awareness in both the pregnant woman and in the womb child, with recognition of women's rights and infants' rights to a humane and holistic birth experience.

New childbirth options, encouraged by changes in medical science, have been refined in recent years and are now ready to be implemented. In the case of Calm Birth, the techniques it uses have been long-revered, and now it is time to put them to use where they are needed probably more than they ever have been. Since two of the three methods in the Calm Birth program come from sacred sources, and the other comes from the genius of American medicine emerging to meet the needs of our times, we have methods that we can respect, methods that can give women profound and healing self-respect. We have benign, risk-free methods available that can make childbirth a process of reengaging the sense of the sacred, while helping women emerge, on a grassroots level, as protectors of the human potential.

Since the Calm Birth method encourages men to participate in the practices with the women, for optimal fetal enhancement, for many men as well as for the women preparing for the event of childbirth, it is an opportunity to transform within. When women and men come together to practice methods to raise the quality of childbirth and the quality of their lives, childbirth becomes a saving grace.

Keys for a New Model of Childbirth Education

Revolutionary childbirth. Meditation may be the only revolution. It is a method that helps people intentionally shift states of being, to come closer to their full potential. Transformational practices take time, but they bring us to our inherent freedom from time. Childbirth meditation frees women into a new domain.

Fearless awareness. Awareness is to be protected as the essence of the quality of life, and women are to be encouraged to have no fear of being completely aware, completely open, fearless to be in union with their all-knowing, unchanging essence. Such awareness is the sanity of primordial health.

A new vision of childbirth anatomy is available to be used. Integrating the vividly alive energy body inseparable from the physical body calls for greater wisdom about the stages of embryo genesis and prenatal development and reverence for sacred knowledge that still comes to us from the past, showing us, as if for the first time, the great potential of capability and function in childbirth. With rediscovered reverence for the preciousness of the human body and its potential, childbirth science and education can begin to appreciate the many dimensions of the nature of life in human birth.

Sacred reality. A true key to appropriate childbirth education is the atmosphere of the sacred and the experience of the miracle of life. This is best engendered by a circle of wise women/childbirth professionals given increasing authority to teach pregnant women and women who plan to become pregnant how to become empowered and realize life in giving birth.

Intention. Because of media communications and because of the advancing perspective of history, the average person has an unavoidable view of the whole planet. Women can learn to practice childbirth methods with the intention to benefit all life. They can learn to intend the advancement of the paradigm of childbirth to benefit the planet. Intention is a powerful resource for childbirth. Women can intend to benefit the world in giving birth and actually do that because intention has unlimited and marvelous potential. Intention to rise above personal limitations and act for the benefit of the world in childbirth may be a vital key to a new model of childbirth.

Sacred sex. Until the last stage of the 20th century the teachings and methods of sexual *tantra*, sacred sex, were carefully guarded secrets of great teaching lineages, particularly the *Nyingma* lineage of Tibetan Buddhism. Though books have been published by people who have accessed some information, it is time for authentic transmission of the vision of sacred sex in childbirth education, for men and woman, so that they may understand the preciousness of the human sexual essences and why they have long been known to be sacred.

The source and potential of life. *Vajrayana* Buddhist experience states that the ever-present primordial ground of awareness is unchanging and unmoving. Timeless. The Zen *koan* "Show me your face before you were born" has been effective for centuries because there is practical access to the primordial source of life. There is a proverb that says something like, "To not know what happened before you were born is to always be a child." That has been remembered and repeated because it is true. If the above teachings are made integral to a new model of childbirth education, people will be guided to know more of what the source and potential of life really are and will be more prepared to know what is born when a child is born.

Afterword

Space of Divinity

By Ruth L. Miller, Ph.D.

A Cultural Context for Childbirth

THOUGH MOST AMERICANS TODAY assume all babies are born in hospitals, such was not the case a few decades ago, and still is not the case in many other countries—most of which have better infant health statistics than ours. Billions of strong women, over millions of years of humanity, have birthed healthy children at home, or in the home of a trusted friend, with the help of women who know and love them and understand the birthing process. Or they have chosen a sacred place to bear their child, outside, apart from other people, moving and massaging their bodies and chanting in ways that ensure an easy birth and a healthy child, having been guided to do so by the skillful and understanding wise women of their community.

Such patterns were the norm in Western culture until the Inquisition killed off millions of women who worked as midwives and healers in Europe and America, and replaced them with a few thousand male physicians and surgeons whose primary experience was with the wounded on battlefields. Then, for the first time, "childbirth blood poisoning" and related conditions were encountered. Lack of controls for infection caused the deaths of thousands of mothers in hospitals and homes. As a result, pregnancy became known as a dangerous "condition," requiring significant medical intervention by trained physicians to ensure the health of mother and child. Progress in the medical specialty of childbirth, called obstetrics, became defined as finding ways to help "weak" women go through a painful process without feeling it, and to remove the infant as quickly as possible from the birth canal. And so we have been taught, for several generations.

The creation of separate birthing centers, the encouragement of nurse-midwives, and the inclusion of family members during labor have gone a long way toward creating a supportive environment for the birthing process, but even they function within the medical model of pregnancy and birth. And the statistics, though far better than a century ago, are still dismal. Too many women come into the childbirth experience totally unprepared—emotionally, physically, or spiritually—for the challenge they will face. They have been disempowered and frightened, and the consequences are, too often, disastrous.

The Wise Woman Tradition

FROM THE MOST ANCIENT TIMES, the mystery of pregnancy and birth has been the central core of spiritual inquiry. From the first awareness of movement of the child within, awe and wonder at the possibility of new life—of creation out of seemingly nothing—fill the mind and heart.

> Woman's awe at her capacity to create life is the basis of mystery. Earliest religious images show pregnancy, rather than birth or nurturing, as *the numinous* or *magical state*.... figurines of women representing the pregnant Goddess go back over thirty thousand years (Monica Sjöö and Barbara Mor, *The Great Cosmic Mother: Rediscovering the Religion of the Earth*, 1987, p. 71).

> Not only is the place of childbirth the sacral place of female life in early cultures ... the mysterious occurrence of men-

> struation and pregnancy and the dangerous episode of child-bearing make it necessary for the inexperienced women to be initiated by those who are informed in the matters (Erich Neumann, *The Great Mother: Analysis of an Archetype,* 1955, p. 159).

Western culture has evolved many new forms since those ancient days, and humanity's early devotion to the Great Mother has been largely replaced by worship of an all-powerful Father. Yet there are hints in the historical documents that, behind the public scenes, in the homes and temples of the women, the old traditions continued. We read in Jeremiah (c. 700 B.C.E. how the women "still weep for Tammuz," the goddess consort, whose death and resurrection were acted out in ancient Sumeria (c. 3500 B.C.E.) and are, even today, part of the annual agricultural cycle in the Middle East. We read Moses' description of Miriam leading the people in a sacred song of celebration after their successful exodus from Egypt, and of her leadership in the wilderness, suggesting that she was a great Wise Woman among the Hebrews. Even her name suggests it: the Hebrew word MRM has two roots: one is related to myrrh, used to anoint the dead (which only women may do in Hebrew culture), and means bitter; the other means height, or greatness.

Miriam, in the Greek form of her name, Mary, appears again in the New Testament. Six Marys are described as associated with Jesus. They came from different towns, they were free to travel about the country with Jesus and his disciples, and they were the ones who kept the men supplied. Clearly, the Miriams were strong, independent women (which is one of the definitions of the word often translated as *virgin*). One of them, Jesus' mother, is called the "Queen of Heaven," which is an ancient term for the goddess, and reflects a tradition in the lineage of David that the mother of the king reigns with him. Another, the Magdalene (meaning tower), has long been called "Apostle to the Apostles," and is typically portrayed as taller, i.e., "greater," than all the men and women around her in ancient art.

The *Nag Hammadi* codices, found outside a Gnostic monastery in Egypt, describe Miriam the Magdalene as Jesus' consort and the primary interpreter of his teachings. Looking back at the Gospels with this information, a number of scholars have reframed her role in Jesus' life and teachings. There's a growing body of evidence that Miriam the Magdalene was a Wise Woman in the ancient tradition—that she was a representative of the goddess who, in age-old rituals, helped to train and support her generation's Yeshua (a name meaning savior), and as his priestess-bride anointed him in the Hebrew sacred marriage ceremony that David and Solomon experienced. Then, as the Gospels tell us, the Magdalene observed his death and resurrection, restoring her people's faith in the power of Life.

Unfortunately the Miriams and their traditions have not been fully described in the histories. Their existence challenged the idea of an exclusively masculine divinity, and writing was taught to only a few men in service to that divinity. Moreover, as we see in the Middle East today, the public men's culture was truly separate from the hidden women's culture. Still, in their homes, in temples and sacred oracles, and in "red tents" where menstruating women were separated from the men, the ancient Wise Woman traditions were passed on from woman to woman throughout the Roman Empire; any man who wished to be emperor was required to marry the high temple priestess.

However, the Christian church, centered in the masculine-divinity culture, could not allow these traditions to continue. So, from medieval times through the 17th century, millions of women who worked as healers and midwives, or dared learn how to read, were tried for "witchcraft" and executed. Thus the Wise Woman tradition was, tragically, almost entirely eradicated from our culture.

A New Balance

FORTUNATELY, SUCH WAS NOT THE CASE in the cultures of the East. There, spiritual leaders have long recognized what Carl Jung discovered in the mid-20th century: that all consciousness has both male and female aspects. As a result, the Hindu, Buddhist, and Taoist traditions have developed methods that enhance both aspects of each individual's spirit, mind, and body.

For millennia, men and women who wish to experience life more fully have been taught these methods. They have been taught by the living example of their teachers, through personalized exercises, and in the stories of others who have gone before them. These stories describe the experiences of those men and women who, having persevered in their intentions, have achieved their full potential and are now living in service to humanity. In the Hindu tradition, these are "great souls" and "saints." In Buddhism, they are called *Buddhas* and *Bodhisattvas*.

One such being is Tara, a *Bodhisattva* who, the story goes, was once a princess devoted to the spiritual path. When told she must pray to be given a man's form so she could pursue her desire for enlightenment, she replied that the idea of male and female is illusion and that, in truth, there is no distinction between male and female (sounding very like Jesus' statement, "there is no male nor female in the kingdom of heaven"), so she need not give up being a woman to achieve enlightenment and relieve souls of suffering. After years of effort, she accomplished her intention, and relieved millions of people from their suffering.

Tara is a model Wise Woman, the embodiment of our potential as human beings, and essential to all Tibetan spiritual practice, including the Dalai Lama's. Her practice teaches us to breathe effectively, to persist with enthusiasm, and to transform suffering, for ourselves and others, by taking disturbances into the heart with the breath and dissolving them in our energy body. She reflects our potential for a life that is empowered, joy-filled, and compassionate.

The methods taught by the men and women who follow Tara's path form the basis for the Calm Birth program. And, as women use these methods, they are empowered to participate fully in their own birthing process, and to assist others. They begin to experience themselves once more as Wise Women who can guide themselves and others through the miracle of childbirth.

In doing so, they can begin to restore the balance, to reduce the birth trauma for both mother and child, and so enhance the quality of life for all—for generations to come.

Acknowledgments

FIRST AND FOREMOST I wish to express profound gratitude to Chögyam Trungpa Rinpoche and Shenphen Dawa Rinpoche, two of my main teachers. Trungpa Rinpoche transmitted the practice of *Ton Len (Sending and Receiving,* or *Exchanging Oneself for Another)* in 1978, and it became one of the essential practices of my life from that time onward. In the Calm Birth program *Ton Len* is applied to childbirth for the first time in the practice of *Giving and Receiving.* Shenphen Rinpoche transmitted the practice of *Vase Breathing* to various students of his, myself included, for many years, starting in 1981. He authorized me to teach it in 1984. He has supported my use of it in the Calm Birth program, where it is applied to childbirth for the first time as the practice of *Womb Breathing.*

In the first two years of this four-year book project, Whitney Wolf, M.A., then director of the Calm Birth program, was very helpful. In her sincere devotion to the Calm Birth program and the book, she helped me establish the manuscript on the computer as I generated the language, the chapters, and the development. She helped me refine the language of the Calm Birth methods, which had been in development for three years, and she did the voice presentation for the second edition of the prenatal methods (CB2). Her voice is also present in the book in some of the interviews with mothers who gave birth with the Calm Birth methods.

At a pivotal early stage of the book's development, David Chamberlain, Ph.D., began to provide invaluable editorial help and guidance. David had been president of the Association of Prenatal and Perinatal Psychology and Health (APPPAH), an international association of childbirth professionals, psychologists, and researchers intent on improving childbirth practices and health. He is an accomplished writer and editor. His editing of "Toward a New Era of Childbirth Education," and "Childbirth Meditation," for publication in the peer-reviewed APPPAH journal, was pivotal in the development of the book. His foreword to this book is a testament to his understanding and support. I'm deeply grateful for his invaluable help.

When I finally felt that the book was ready for publication, I tried to locate a literary agent. Sally Brady, of Brady Literary Management, expressed keen interest in the book, and thought that a mainstream publisher might be interested. She saw the subjects of the rights of women and infants in childbirth as "hot" issues. Upon careful reading of the manuscript she suggested a large-scale restructuring of the book. My instincts were that her suggestions were appropriate, and I undertook a reworking of the text. Sally is a dedicated Buddhist practitioner. She saw the book as a strong attempt to bring sacred methods into childbirth, where they are profoundly needed.

Even after Sally began to show the book to major publishers, the book had a life of its own, and I continued to work on it. Two of the certified teachers in the Calm Birth program, Catherine Stone, C.D., and Dara Knerr, C.D., proved to be important in helping finish the language. As experienced doulas, with a vested interest in the Calm Birth program, they spontaneously took up the language as their own and suggested valuable improvements throughout, as if women had arisen from the heart of the book to provide touches and statements that needed to come from women.

Ruth L. Miller, Ph.D., has been a great help in preparing the manuscript for publication, and has been another important set of eyes from the present Wise Women, to make sure that the book was right. As the book came to final finish, Ruth was present to influence the final form of the conclusion of the vision of A New Era of Childbirth Education. At my suggestion she wrote an Afterword to the book that adds invaluably to the intention and scope of this work. Ruth's contribution to the book is truly great.

Joan Kalvelage, Ph.D., was helpful in important ways. A psychologist and an experienced meditator, Joan read the book and helped me see that my use of references to meditation science was important and needed to be amplified. She also helped me see a way to present the insights of luminaries of physics in a nontechnical, accessible way.

I'm grateful to JoAnn Walker, R.N. She was the first director of the Calm Birth program and facilitated the first interviews with mothers who gave birth with the Calm Birth methods. The records of those interviews were the first pages of the book to be produced. Donna Worden was also very helpful in the beginning of the program, arranging the very first training seminar and then being the voice on the first audioguide presenting two of the methods in their initial formulation.

Gerald Lehrburger, M.D., senior member of the Calm Birth board of directors, has been an important supporter of the program from the beginning. The Health Research Institute, which he founded and directs, has provided important assistance.

I'm also very grateful to Sandra Bardsley, C.N.M., R.N., C.D., and Colleen Graham, a special childbirth educator. They were both founding members of the Association of Prenatal and Perinatal Psychology and Health and have been invaluable supporters of the Calm Birth program for years. Colleen was on the board of directors for several years. Sandra, a gifted nurse midwife who has birthed more than three thousand children naturally, has been a leading figure in the establishment of doula organizations in America. Sandra made contributions to the refining of the methods for recording and publication, assuring that the accomplished nurse mother was in the voice transmitting the methods. The voice of the medicine woman is clearly in the Calm Birth methods.

Finally, I'm deeply grateful to Richard Grossinger, publisher of North Atlantic Books. Richard is much more than a publisher. His work in embryology and the history of medicine is of great value. In response to this book he called it "very powerful, well-written, and a gift to publish." That was the sign that I'd found the right publisher.

Glossary

Advanced natural childbirth: New childbirth methods in which meditation practices give women empowering means to adhere to and advance the principals of natural childbirth.

Ancient wisdom methods: Various self-development and healing methods from traditional meditation science, proven through ages of use and currently increasingly appreciated by Western science.

Audioguidance: The use of advanced audio technology to guide those who listen to shift into greater function; an advanced basis of discipline.

Chi [Qi]: Vital energy. There is external and internal *chi.* "Chi is fundamental to Chinese medical thinking, yet no one English word or phrase can adequately capture its meaning. Perhaps we can think of Chi as matter on the verge of becoming energy or energy at the point of materializing" (Kaptchuk, 1983, p. 35).

Childbirth meditation: The practice of meditation in prenatal care is a means of enrichment, and in postnatal care it is a valuable self-care method. The methods may be from any one of a number of available traditions of meditation science.

Complementary and Alternative Medicine (CAM): The term for various medical disciplines, mostly traditional, now included in the expanded medical paradigm. Dissatisfaction with conventional medical practices has created great popular interest in and respect for CAM.

Energy medicine: Medical practices where the body is seen to be a body of energy systems and fields; practices of seeing and modifying those fields therapeutically constitutes diagnosis and treatment. Acupuncture, acupressure, bodywork, and conscious breathing are each a kind of energy medicine.

Enriched pregnancy: Childbirth practices, including playing good music, reading to the womb child, and meditation, are used in prenatal care to access the optimal health and developmental potential in childbirth.

Expanded anatomy: The systems of human multidimensional anatomy, the inseparable physical body and energy body, offer a vision of what the body is and what functions may be developed through methods of meditation science.

Fine breathing: Deep breathing that intentionally absorbs vital energy from the air as well as accesses optimal oxygenation.

Giving and Receiving: An advanced natural childbirth method that brings the experience of healing into childbirth. It is valuable in both prenatal and postnatal care.

Hara (Japanese): The vital center; focal point of *Zen* meditation, comparable to and perhaps the same as the *tan tien* in Chinese *Tai Chi* meditation and the Life Vase *(Bum Chung)* in Tibetan *Vajrayana* meditation. It is a receiver for energies breathed into it, for greater function and increase of life force.

Meditation: A consciousness discipline that enables people to experience greater levels of awareness and health, normally blocked by the mind in its undisciplined activity.

Meditation science: The scientific knowledge behind meditation methods from different traditions, with understanding of the short- and long-term effects of the application of those methods. These methods have been tested and proved through centuries of disciplined use, yielding repeatable results.

Mindfulness-Based Stress Reduction (MBSR): The renowned mind/body medicine clinic at the University of Massachusetts Medical Center. Established in 1979, it has trained more than eighteen thousand people in medicine/meditation methods and has been the model for hundreds of such programs established in America, Canada, and Europe.

Mind/body medicine: An important development in the history of medicine, expanding the medical paradigm in the West since the 1970s, in which meditation and other interventions using the mind enable the body to improve its function. Called self-care, it's seen as the heart of a new medical paradigm.

Optimal childbirth breathing: Breathing practice, such as *Womb Breathing*, in which vital energy from the air as well as full oxygenation are breathed, enriching the child with energy and developmental intention.

Paradigm: A pattern, example, or model. A concept accepted by most people in an intellectual community, as those in one of the natural sciences, because it seems to be effective in explaining a complex process, idea, or set of data.

Paradigm shift: A change in the way individuals or cultures see the world, or interpret phenomena, giving people a sense of having new eyes or new knowing. Paradigm shifts are caused by evolutionary progress, setting people free of restrictive conditioning.

Placenta: The soft, spongy organ through which the woman's blood nourishes the fetus, through the umbilical cord; it is expelled after birth, sometimes treated as sacred and buried as such. In optimal birth the umbilical cord is not cut as long as it is pulsing oxygen and nourishment to the child, which could be for an hour or more.

Practice of Opening: An advanced natural childbirth method using a reclining progressive relaxation technique. Those who do the practice are brought into life force in their cellular nature in various ways, resulting in nervous system healing, increased knowledge of the body and its capabilities, and direct developmental connection with the womb child.

Prana (Sanskrit): A subtle but powerful life energy pervading all matter; universal life force. Probably the same as *chi*. Current science refers to it as universal energy and speaks of its field being measurable. It can be breathed and utilized, as in the practice of *Womb Breathing.*

Shamatha (Sanskrit): Calm abiding. A meditation practice for calming down and staying calm in order to rest free of the disturbances of the mind. Various concentration techniques are used. The most common is following the breath.

Slow breathing: Deep, abdominal breathing becomes slow breathing, healthier breathing using minimal energy. Ancient wisdom says that each life has a certain amount of breaths to live, and intentionally slow breathing brings long life.

Subtle body: Inner body, or energy body. Traditionally esoteric systems envisioned several bodies inherent in the physical body. Sometimes called astral, mental, and causal bodies, these bodies have been seen to be operating at successively higher frequencies than the physical body. They are engaged, activated, and utilized by evolutionary work. Medicine today accepts the presence of an energy body in the physical body, in which subtle body functions are integral to physical functions.

Tan tien: Focal point for *Tai Chi* meditation, situated in the navel center. The *tan tien* is similar to the Life Vase and the *Hara,* and may be the same.

Umbilicus: The depression in the center of the abdomen where the umbilical cord has been cut; the navel.

Vajrayana (Sanskrit): The Diamond Vehicle; the Buddhism of Tibet; the ultimate stage of the development of the Buddha's teachings. Based on the vow of compassionate service to all life, *Vajrayana* Buddhism is known for its variety of profound methods.

Vase Breathing: This practice, a treasure of ancient wisdom, is characterized by breathing vital essence from the air down into the Life Vase, *Bum Chung* (Tibetan), in the navel center, which feeds the energy up into the central psychic channel for greater function.

Vipashyana (Sanskrit): Clear or wider seeing; panoramic awareness; extraordinary insight; "Wisdom Mind" arising from *shamatha* practice.

Visualization: Most often a concentration method in which the whole body, a specific body system, or a body process is envisioned purposefully, to alter the body's biology beneficially. To be most successful visualization should be based on calming meditation.

Wise Woman tradition: The ancient understanding that in every community there were women who held and shared the wisdom of previous generations for the well-being of all. They were healers, teachers, midwives, and coordinators of community-wide events and ceremonies. They participated with other elders in decision-making for the community. Historically in Western culture a Wise Woman was in charge of the main temple. She married the king and co-ruled with him.

Womb Breathing: A method of advanced natural childbirth developed from traditional meditation science. Using a new vision of the body of the pregnant woman, extending childbirth anatomy, this deep breathing practice gives women an expanded sense of their natural birthing capabilities.

World Health Organization (WHO): The international health and research services of the United Nations.

Yoga: Literally "union." Originally a general category for various kinds of meditation practice, today in the West yoga usually refers to *hatha yoga*, stretching and breathing exercises, which can be beneficial in prenatal care.

Zygote: The union of male and female reproductive cells that develops into a new individual.

References

Preface

Benson, H. (1996). *Timeless Healing: The Power and Biology of Belief.* New York, NY: Simon & Schuster.

Bradley, R. (1965). *Husband-Coached Childbirth.* New York, NY: Harper & Row.

Dick-Read, G. (1944). *Childbirth without Fear.* New York, NY: Harper & Row.

Dossey, L. (1993). *Healing Words: The Power of Prayer and the Practice of Medicine.* San Francisco, CA: HarperCollins.

Ferguson, M. (1980). *The Aquarian Conspiracy.* Los Angeles, CA: J. P. Tarcher, Inc.

Shealy, C. N., and Myss, C. (1993). *The Creation of Health.* Walpole, NH: Stillpoint Publications.

Wagner, M. (1994). *The Birth Machine: The Search for Appropriate Birth Technology.* Camperdown, Australia: ACE Graphics.

I. Background

Achterberg, J. (1990). *Woman as Healer.* Boston, MA: Shambhala Publications.

II. Childbirth Meditation

Astin, A., et al, (1987). *An Analysis of Coping.* Los Angeles, CA: Higher Education Research Institute, University of California.

Benson, H. (1996). *Timeless Healing: The Power and Biology of Belief.* New York, NY: Simon & Schuster.

Borysenko, J., and Borysenko, M. (1994). *The Power of the Mind to Heal.* Carson, CA: Hay House.

Brennan, B. (1993). *Light Emerging.* New York, NY: Bantam Books.

Cardoso, R., et al. (2004). "Meditation in Health: An Operational Definition." *Brain Research Protocols* 14(1): 58–60. www.elsevier.com/locate/brainresprot

Chang, G. C. C. (1963). *The Six Yogas of Naropa.* Ithaca, NY: Snow Lion Publications.

Chopra, D. (1990). *Quantum Healing: Exploring the Frontiers of Mind/Body Medicine.* New York, NY: Bantam Books.

Davis-Floyd, R. (2003). *Birth as an American Rite of Passage.* Berkeley, CA: University of California Press.

Dossey, L. (1993). *Healing Words: The Power of Prayer and the Practice of Medicine.* San Francisco, CA: HarperCollins.

Hopper, J. (1989). "Ommm ... Please Pass the DHEA." *Health* 21: 34.

Jacobson, E. (1938). *Progressive Relaxation.* Chicago, IL: University of Chicago Press.

Kabat-Zinn, J. (1990). *Full Catastrophe Living: Using the Wisdom of Your Body and Mind to Face Stress, Pain, and Illness.* New York, NY: Bantam Doubleday Dell.

Kabat-Zinn, J., et al. (1995). "Meditation, Melatonin and Breast/Prostate Cancer." *Medical Hypotheses* 44: 39–46.

Khalsa, D. S. (2001). *Meditation as Medicine.* New York, NY: Simon & Schuster.

Murphy, M., and Donovan, S. (1999). *The Physical and Psychological Effects of Meditation: A Review of Contemporary Research with a Comprehensive Bibliography.* Sausalito, CA: Institute of Noetic Sciences.

Myss, C. (1996). *Anatomy of the Spirit.* New York, NY: Crown Publishers.

Odent, M. (1994). *Birth Reborn.* Medford, NJ: Birth Works Press.

Pert, C. (1997). *Molecules of Emotion.* New York, NY: Simon & Schuster.

Pierpaoli, W., and Regelson, W. (1995). *The Melatonin Miracle.* New York, NY: Simon & Schuster.

Reiter, R., and Robinson, J. (1995). *Melatonin: Your Body's Natural*

Wonder Drug. New York, NY: Bantam Books.

Sogyal Rinpoche. (1993). *The Tibetan Book of Living and Dying*. San Francisco, CA: HarperSanFrancisco.

Tsai, S. (1993). "The Effects of Relaxation Training, Combining Meditation and Guided Imagery, on Self-Perceived Stress among Chinese Nurses in Large Teaching Hospitals in Taiwan, ROC." *Dissertation Abstracts International* 53, no. 8–B.m.

Wagner, M. (1994). *The Birth Machine: The Search for Appropriate Birth Technology*. Camperdown, Australia: ACE Graphics.

III. Childbirth and Energy Medicine

Baker, J. P. (1974). *Prenatal Yoga and Natural Childbirth*. Berkeley, CA: North Atlantic Books.

Brennan, B. (1988). *Hands of Light*. New York, NY: Bantam Books.

Lamaze, F. (1958). *Painless Childbirth: The Lamaze Method*. New York, NY: Simon & Schuster.

Leboyer, F. (1975). *Birth without Violence*. New York, NY: Alfred A. Knopf, Inc.

Leboyer, F. (1978). *Inner Beauty, Inner Light: Yoga for Pregnant Women*. New York, NY: Newmarket Press.

Myss, C. (1996). *Anatomy of the Spirit*. New York, NY: Harmony Books.

Ornish, D. (1990). *Program for Reversing Heart Disease*. New York, NY: Random House.

Oschman, J. (2000). *Energy Medicine*. Edinburgh, Scotland: Harcourt Publisher.

IV. Pregnancy as Master Path

Castaneda, C. (1998). *Magical Passes*. New York, NY: HarperCollins.

Ch'ing, C. M. (1985). *Cheng Tzu's Thirteen Treatises on T'ai Chi Ch'uan*. Berkeley, CA: North Atlantic Books.

Kaptchuk, T. (1983). *The Web That Has No Weaver*. New York, NY: Congdon & Weed.

Montagu, A. (1954). *The Natural Superiority of Women*. New York,

NY: The MacMillan Company.

Pert, C. (1997). *Molecules of Emotion.* New York, NY: Simon & Schuster.

Tolle, E. (1999). *The Power of Now.* Novato, CA: New World Library.

Von Durckheim, K. G. (1977). *Hara.* London, England: George Allen & Unwin, Ltd.

Wilhelm, R. (1955). *The Secret of the Golden Flower.* New York, NY: Wehman Bros.

Zenji, H. (1963). *The Embossed Tea Kettle.* London, England: George Allen & Unwin, Ltd.

V. The Calm Birth Methods

Castaneda, C. (1998). *Magical Passes.* New York, NY: HarperCollins.

Hayward, J., and Hayward, K. (2001). *Sacred World.* Boston, MA: Shambhala Publications.

Khalsa, D. S., and Stauth, C. (2001). *Meditation as Medicine.* New York, NY: Simon & Schuster.

Hendricks, G. (1995). *Conscious Breathing: Breathwork for Health, Stress Release, and Personal Mastery.* New York, NY: Simon and Schuster.

Leonard, G., and Murphy, M. (1995). *The Life We Are Given.* New York, NY: Tarcher/Putnam.

Montagu, A. (1954). *The Natural Superiority of Women.* New York, NY: The MacMillan Company.

Myss, C. (1996). *Anatomy of the Spirit.* New York, NY: Crown Publishers.

Northrup, Christiane. (1998). *Women's Bodies, Women's Wisdom.* New York, NY: Bantam Books.

Odent, M. (1994). *Birth Reborn.* Medford, NJ: Birth Works Press.

Pelletier, K. (1977). *Mind as Slayer, Mind as Healer.* New York, NY: Dell Publishing.

Rama, S. (1979). *Science of Breath.* Honesdale, PA: The Himalayan International Institute of Yogic Science and Philosophy.

VI. Eight Calm Births

Gaskin, I. M. (2003). *Ina May's Guide to Childbirth.* New York, NY: Bantam/Dell.

Sogyal Rinpoche. (1994). *The Tibetan Book of Living and Dying.* San Francisco, CA: HarperSanFrancisco.

VII. New Childbirth Medicine

Chamberlain, D. (1998). *The Mind of Your Newborn Baby.* Berkeley, CA: North Atlantic Books.

Chamberlain, D. (1999). "Selected Works by David Chamberlain." *Journal of Prenatal and Perinatal Psychology and Health* 14(1–2): 1–194.

Grof, S. (1993). *The Holotropic Mind.* New York, NY: HarperCollins.

Hallett, E. (1995). *Soul Trek: Meeting Our Children on the Way to Birth.* Hamilton, MT: Light Hearts Publishing.

Jacobson, E. (1938). *Progressive Relaxation.* Chicago, IL: University of Chicago Press.

Kabat-Zinn, J. (1990). *Full Catastrophe Living: Using the Wisdom of Your Body and Mind to Face Stress, Pain, and Illness.* New York, NY: Bantam Doubleday Dell.

Murphy, M., and Donovan, S. (1999). *The Physical and Psychological Effects of Meditation: A Review of Contemporary Research with a Comprehensive Bibliography.* Sausalito, CA: Institute of Noetic Sciences.

Schwartz, F. (1997). "Prenatal Stress Reduction, Music and Medical Cost Savings." *Journal of Prenatal and Perinatal Psychology and Health* 12(1): 1–44.

Wilber, K. (1999). *The Marriage of Sense and Soul.* Boston, MA: Shambhala Publications.

VIII. Toward a New Era of Childbirth Education

Benson, H. (1996). *Timeless Heaing: The Power and Biology of Belief.* New York, NY: Simon & Schuster.

Bohm, D. (1980). *Wholeness and the Implicate Order.* London, England: Routledge.

Bradley, R. (1965). *Husband-Coached Childbirth.* New York, NY: Harper & Row.

Chamberlain, D. (1998). *The Mind of Your Newborn Baby.* Berkeley, CA: North Atlantic Books.

Chamberlain, D. (1999). "Selected Works by David Chamberlain." *Journal of Prenatal and Perinatal Psychology and Health* 14(1–2): 1–194.

Chopra, D. (1990). *Quantum Healing: Exploring the Frontiers of Mind/Body Medicine.* New York, NY: Bantam Books.

Davis-Floyd, R. (2003). *Birth as an American Rite of Passage.* Berkeley, CA: University of California Press.

Dick-Read, G. (1944). *Childbirth without Fear.* New York, NY: Harper & Row.

Dossey, L. (1989). *Recovering the Soul.* New York, NY: Bantam Books.

Dossey, L. (1993). *Healing Words: The Power of Prayer and the Practice of Medicine.* New York, NY: HarperCollins.

Einstein, A. (1954). *Ideas and Opinions.* New York, NY: Crown Publishing.

Ferguson, M. (1980). *The Aquarian Conspiracy.* Los Angeles, CA: J. P. Tarcher, Inc.

Grof, S. (1993). *The Holotropic Mind: The Three Levels of Consciousness and How They Shape Our Lives.* New York, NY: HarperCollins.

Hallett, E. (1995). *Soul Trek: Meeting Our Children on the Way to Birth.* Hamilton, MT: Light Hearts Publishing.

James, W. (1961). *Varieties of Religious Experience.* New York, NY: Collier.

Journal of Prenatal and Perinatal Psychology and Health. (1986–2005). Forestville, CA: APPPAH.

Lamaze, F. (1958). *Painless Childbirth: The Lamaze Method.* New York, NY: Simon & Schuster.

Leonard, G., and Murphy, M. (1995). *The Life We Are Given.* New York, NY: Tarcher/Putnam.

Margenau, H. (1987). *The Miracle of Existence.* Boston, MA: New Science Library.

Odent, M. (1994). *Birth Reborn.* Medford, NJ: Birth Works Press.

Rosen, S. (1997). *The Reincarnation Controversy: Uncovering the Truth in the World Religions.* Badger, CA: Torchlight Publishing, Inc.

Schrodinger, E. (1969). *What Is Life?* and *Mind and Matter.* London, England: Cambridge University Press.

Shealy, C. N., and Myss, C. (1993). *The Creation of Health.* Walpole, NH: Stillpoint Publishing.

Tarthang Tulku. (2002). *Mind over Matter.* Berkeley, CA: Dharma Publishing.

Verny, T. (1981). *The Secret Life of the Unborn Baby.* New York, NY: Dell Publishing Co.

Verny, T. (2002). *Tomorrow's Baby: The Art and Science of Parenting from Conception Through Infancy.* New York, NY: Simon & Schuster.

Wagner, M. (1994). *The Birth Machine: The Search for Appropriate Birth Technology.* Camperdown, Australia: ACE Graphics.

Wilber, K. (2002). *Boomeritis.* Boston, MA: Shambhala Publications.

About the Author

Robert Newman has been developing and implementing programs in the medical uses of meditation for the past fifteen years. He is the primary developer and teacher of the Calm Birth methods, and is currently training the teachers who will carry the program forward. In 2001 Mr. Newman published his first book, *Disciples of the Buddha: Living Images of Meditation,* with an introduction by Chögyam Trungpa Rinpoche, and based on photographic studies of some of the most important works of art ever made, art revealing the nature of meditation. That book represents his early work with meditation masters of Tibet, teachers who are the source of the methods he learned and has applied in the medical establishment. Mr. Newman's third book, *Calm Healing: The Medical Uses of Meditation,* which will be published by North Atlantic Books in 2006, presents his proprietary methods for heart care, cancer care, Alzheimer's care, near-death care, and other areas of medicine.

David B. Chamberlain, Ph.D., is a California psychologist, teacher at the Santa Barbara Graduate Institute, and author of more than fifty publications including *The Mind of Your Newborn Baby* (North Atlantic Books, 1998), now in its third edition in ten languages.

Ruth L. Miller, Ph.D., is author of *150 Years of Healing* (Abib, 2000) and *Unveiling Your Hidden Power* (forthcoming). She has degrees in anthropology, cybernetics, and the systems sciences, and teaches metaphysics and "New Paradigms of Science and Spirituality" at New West Seminary in Oregon City, Oregon. Dr. Miller serves on the board of MediGrace, Inc., the nonprofit corporation that offers the Calm Birth program.

About Calm Birth

For information about the Calm Birth program, products, and services, please visit the Calm Birth web site: www.CalmBirth.org

About MediGrace

For information about the MediGrace products for cancer care, cardiovascular care, HIV-AIDS care, Alzheimer's care, and near-death care, please visit the MediGrace web site: www.MediGrace.org

Also available from North Atlantic Books

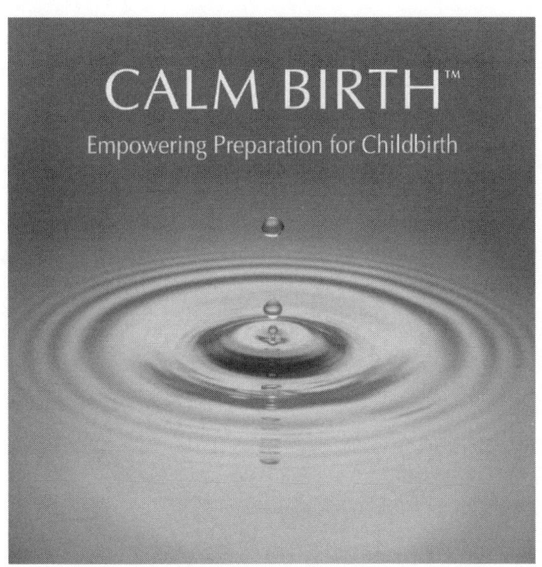

Calm Birth CD

Empowering Preparation for Childbirth

1. *Practice of Opening:* 22:15 minutes

2. *Womb Breathing:* 22:12 minutes

3. *Giving and Receiving:* 12:21 minutes

Text: Robert Bruce Newman

Voice: Dara Knerr

Music: Michael Mish

$19.95 • ISBN 1-55643-588-6

www.northatlanticbooks.com
orders@northatlanticbooks.com
1-800-337-2665